GILLES DE LA TOURETTE'S SYNDROME

Volume 1

INTERNATIONAL REGISTRY

edited by

F. S. Abuzzahab Sr., M.D., Ph.D.
Clinical Associate Professor
Departments of Psychiatry, Pharmacology
and Family Practice and Community Health
University of Minnesota

and

F. O. Anderson, M.D.
Resident in Psychiatry
University of Minnesota

Supported in part by Psychopharmacology Fund, Minnesota Medical Foundation, and Work Study Program of the University of Minnesota, Minneapolis, Minnesota 55455

International Standard Book Number: 0-917126-00-9

Library of Congress Catalog Card Number: 76-9663

Printed in the United States of America

MASON PUBLISHING COMPANY

802 Finch Building
St. Paul, Minnesota 55101
U.S.A.

To our patients, who are our best teachers.

CONTRIBUTING AUTHORS

F.S. Abuzzahab Sr., M.D., Ph.D.
Box 393 Mayo
University of Minnesota Hospitals
Minneapolis, MN 55455 U.S.A.

Floyd O. Anderson, M.D.
Box 393 Mayo
University of Minnesota Hospitals
Minneapolis, MN 55455 U.S.A.

Wlodzimierz Borak, M.D.
Hospital for Nervous Diseases
Gniezno, Poland

John A. Corbett, M.R.C.P., D.C.H., D.P.M.
Maudsley Hospital
Denmark Hill
London S.E. 5, England

S.J.M. Fernando, M.A., M.B., B.Ch., D.P.M.
Claybury Hospital
Woodford Bridge
Essex, England

Barry N. Fine, M.D.
Department of Psychiatry
University of Iowa
Iowa City, IA 52240 U.S.A.

Marie Fisarova, C.Sc.
Department of Neurology
Okresni Ustav Narodniho Zdravi
Strakonice, Czechoslovakia

Donald A. Galbraith, M.D.
Children's Psychiatric Institute
University of Western Ontario
London, Ontario, Canada

Evelyn P. Heimlich, Research Assistant
New York State Psychiatric Institute
722 W. 168th Street
New York, NY 10032 U.S.A.

Laszlo Ivan, M.D.
Second Clinic of Neurology and Psychiatry
Medical University
Budapest, Hungary

Richard L. Jenkins, M.D.
Department of Psychiatry
University of Iowa
Iowa City, IA 52240 U.S.A.

Walter Knopp, M.D.
Ohio State University
College of Medicine
Columbus, Ohio 43210 U.S.A.

Elzbieta Koprowska-Milewska, M.D.
Szpitala dla Nerwowo i Psychicznie Chorych
Katowice, ul.
Bankowa 27/79, Poland

J.M. Leger, M.D.
Service de Psychiatrie
Centre Hospitalier Regional
Limoges, France

Alexander R. Lucas, M.D.
Child and Adolescent Psychiatry
Mayo Clinic
Rochester, MN 55901 U.S.A.

Doris H. Milman, M.D.
Department of Pediatrics
State University of New York
Brooklyn, NY 11203 U.S.A.

Mary C. MacKay, M.D.
New York State Psychiatric Institute
722 W. 168th Street
New York, NY 10032 U.S.A.

Ewa Osetowska, M.D.
Institute of Comparative Neuropathology
Centre of Experimental and Clinical Medicine
Polish Academy of Sciences
Gniezno, Poland

Yves Ranty, M.D.
Service de Psychiatrie
Centre Hospitalier Regional
Limoges, France

Libuse Richterova, M.D.
Prague 5, Kartouzska 14
Czechoslovakia

Jean-Noel Seignot, M.D.
32, Boulevard LaFayette
62-Calais, France

Vicdan A. Senler, M.D.
2007 Lakeland Road
Anchorage, KY 40223 U.S.A.

K. Singer, M.B., M.R.C.P.E., D.P.M.
Hong Kong Psychiatric Centre
High Street, Hong Kong

Marilyn Strayer, M.D.
Ohio State University
College of Medicine
Columbus, Ohio 43210 U.S.A.

Timothy Turner, M.D.
Department of Psychiatry
Victoria Hospital
University of Western Ontario
London, Ontario, Canada

TABLE OF CONTENTS

TABLE OF CONTENTS

TABLE OF CONTENTS

Preface

My interest in this esoteric disorder goes back to my medical school years when my dynamic mentor, Dr. A. S. Drooby, touched on this disorder in one of his lectures at the American University of Beirut, Beirut, Republic of Lebanon. I furtively looked into the corners of the psychiatric hospital during my medical student clerkship for a clinical case, but my search was to no avail and the disorder remained dormant in my memory, for a few years.

It surfaced again when I saw my first case during my residency at the Henry Phipps Psychiatric Clinic of the Johns Hopkins Hospital, Baltimore, Maryland. Dr. Eduard Ascher, my teacher, rekindled my interest in this disorder by his exciting lectures and its possible connection with more esoteric disorders such as myriachit and latah. As I recall, the cases at Phipps suffering from this disorder were museum pieces, since they were there for teaching purposes and as far as treatment was concerned their condition remained unhalted.

Following a stint in Graduate School in pharmacology, I resumed clinical work and was fascinated by the reports that haloperidol (Haldol) was able to control the symptoms of this disorder. This opened the door for more cases to come to the recognition of physicians since treatment is now available. However, the natural history of this disorder remained shrouded with many uncertainties. One single investigator was unable to generate enough cases to reach definitive conclusions. In addition, it was not known if haloperidol (Haldol) should be continued throughout the life of the patient or whether it should be stopped when the symptoms are controlled, what happens to the untreated patients, and a myriad of other questions which were being raised and for which no answer was available.

The International Registry of Gilles de la Tourette's Syndrome was launched at that time to find answers to some of those questions and help the unfortunate ones afflicted with this disorder. The success of haloperidol (Haldol) also opened the door to the possibility of verifying the neurochemical lesion of this disorder. I did speculate about such a possibility in an abstract submitted to the American Psychiatric Association's Annual Meeting in 1968, but although the abstract was rejected, there was further confirmation of this possibility by the later work of Dr. Messiha and the speculations by Dr. Solomon Snyder.

This book represents the first volume of a series of publications on this disorder. We have tried to focus on the results of our International Registry. The first section comprises the papers presented in the panel on the International Registry of Gilles de la Tourette's Syndrome at the American Psychiatric Association Meeting. The second section is devoted to papers from other investigators who were unable to attend the panel discussions. Current knowledge about the disorder is summarized in the third section. An alphabetical bibliography of 508 references constitutes the final section.

Volume 2 will be devoted to English translations of papers of Bouteille, Itard, Charcot, Gilles de la Tourette, Guinon and Catrou, who helped delineate this diagnositc entity.

The third volume will be devoted to New Vistas on Gilles de la Tourette's Syndrome. The papers have been submitted as a symposium to be held in conjunction with the World Congress of Psychiatry, Honolulu, Hawaii, U.S.A., August 1977.

Finally, thoughts are being devoted to a Centennial Celebration of the publication of Gilles de la Tourette, to be held at the Salpetriere, Paris, France, 1985.

The publication of this volume and the preparations of future volumes would not have been possible without the able assistance of Dianne Dvorak, Sara Hunter, Mary Sherman and Terry Yuretich.

April, 1976 F. S. Abuzzahab Sr.

INTRODUCTION

Eduard Ascher, M.D.
Associate Professor of Psychiatry,
The Johns Hopkins University School of Medicine
Associate Clinical Professor of Psychiatry,
University of Maryland School of Medicine
Baltimore, MD 21205 U.S.A.

In recent years there has been increasing interest in this syndrome named after Gilles de la Tourette who wrote the first comprehensive treatise on the subject.

There are a number of reasons to explain this development. First of all, it has a highly phonetic, even exotic name. Also Gilles de la Tourette was still a student when he made his brilliant observations and recorded them. Yet, the most striking features are the sequence and nature of the symptoms which occur with such amazing regularity in patients all over the globe that this factor alone was considered to indicate the presence of organic brain disease.

Few syndromes in psychiatry lend themselves so well to a study of the interplay of psychological with organic factors. Can coprolalia be understood in terms of damage to cells of the basal ganglia? Is the vocal tic the result of habit spasms or evidence of disturbance in brain metabolism? The authors of this book were fully aware that only a compilation of data and pooling of experiences would eventually provide answers to these questions. It was with this aim in mind that they established an International Registry and now present the collected papers in book form. The reader is also brought up to date on the most recent developments especially as they pertain to treatment of this syndrome which was once thought to inevitably lead to insanity.

This book is just a beginning. It should encourage all those interested in this condition to keep up their professional contact with each other through reporting of new cases and exchange of views in international seminars.

The authors deserve all the support and gratitude for having made this possible through the Registry and this volume.

SECTION ONE: PANEL PAPERS ON INTERNATIONAL REGISTRY OF GILLES de la TOURETTE'S SYNDROME HELD DURING THE AMERICAN PSYCHIATRIC ASSOCIATION 123rd ANNUAL MEETING 1970

SAN FRANCISCO, CALIFORNIA

Gilles de la Tourette's Syndrome. Volume 1: International Registry, p. 3-5, edited by F. Abuzzahab Sr. and F. Anderson. Mason Publishing Co., St. Paul ©1976.

GILLES DE LA TOURETTE'S SYNDROME

J. A. Corbett, M.R.C.P., D.C.H., D.P.M.
Maudsley Hospital
Denmark Hill
London S.E. 5 England

Although a number of case studies and reviews of Tourette's syndrome have been published, various issues remain to be resolved, including: (1) the need to reach some agreement on the diagnostic criteria, (2) the pathology of the condition, (3) the prognosis, and (4) the optimal treatment. These problems might be more easily resolved with an international study based on larger numbers of cases than so far published.

A number of studies carried out at Maudsley Hospital over the past five years give some indication of the way in which these issues might be re-examined.[99 101 102] These investigations were initiated by an interest in the treatment both of this condition, and of the tic syndrome as a whole, with haloperidol, which arose from the work of Jenkins and his colleagues and of Lucas.[85 88 282 283 284 286] A large scale follow-up study of tics and Gilles de la Tourette's syndrome[101] and also photographic and neurophysiological studies[102] were undertaken, leading to the conclusion that the importance of the syndrome as a psychosomatic phenomenon outweighs its rarity. Moreover, it is one of the few well-defined conditions which clearly spans childhood, adolescence, and adulthood and provides a link among these areas of development.

It seems likely that Tourette's syndrome is not etiologically distinct from other manifestations of the tic syndrome except in its severity and in the interesting development of coprolalia. Basically the syndrome seems to be a distortion of a normal developmental phenomenon, the startle reaction, which is the motor response to a sudden, powerful stimulus (*e.g.*, a gun shot) described in detail 30 years ago by Landis and Hunt.[265] These deductions arise from the following findings:

1. The association of tics with other developmental abnormalities — for example, the preponderance in males, the association with other habit disorders, and the age and mode of onset.[101]
2. The similarity of the tic movements and even the vocalizations to those seen in the startle response demonstrated by high speed cinephotography.[102]
3. The strong similarity in the distribution, mode of spread, and progression of the movements in the startle reaction and tic syndrome (*ie.*, eyeblink occurring first and more frequently, with progression of movements down the body and improvement in the converse direction).[101 102]
4. The tendency of the startle response to behave as a conditioned reflex,[265] and also the response of tics to behavior therapy (for example, massed practice).[94 95 163 379 375 493]
5. The finding that a similar galvanic skin response occurs following both tics and the startle response.[102]

It seems very probable that tics are reinforced by parental and personal anxiety. We found a very high rate of affective illness in mothers of children with tics and Tourette's syndrome, double the rate of psychiatric consultation in mothers of children attending the Maudsley Hospital

Children's Department with nonorganic emotional disorders.

Of 180 patients with tics and Tourette's syndrome attending Maudsley over the past 20 years, 23% had suffered from vocal tics at some time and, in 12% of these, the vocal tics were the only symptoms. Multiple tics were present in 50% of cases.

In the follow-up of 89 patients in whom tics were the main complaint, only 20% of 18 with only vocal tics recovered completely, whereas 50% of those with nonvocal tics did so. Although all those with coprolalia improved, none recovered completely. While the tics improved, there was a marked tendency for anxiety and other psychiatric symptoms to persist in the tiqueurs.

The mode of development of simple vocal tics into coprolalia must remain speculative, but the most attractive hypothesis is that of MacDonald[289] based on a cybernetics model. He suggested that vocal tics, which often resemble monosyllabic swear words, become shaped into actual words by a feedback mechanism, and this may be facilitated by emotions of hostility and aggression in adolescence. This hypothesis is particularly apt if one considers tics to be an alternative mode of affective expression as suggested by our data, which show a low correlation with symptoms involving overt aggression such as fighting and temper outbursts, but a higher one with depression, obsessional symptoms, and hypochondriasis.

Thus, as with other developmental disorders, tics in Gilles de la Tourette's syndrome may be incorporated into the psychopathology of the individual. This usually first occurs in adolescence. Increasing emotional disturbance at this period may be seen in other developmental disorders such as encopresis and also, for example, with severe reading disability. It seems possible that the symptoms of echolalia and echopraxia may acquire symbolic significance at adolescence, although I doubt if this occurs earlier, as psychoanalytic writers have suggested.[164 260 317]

Treatment should be directed at interfering with this reinforcing process by means of such methods as drugs, the most useful of which seem to be haloperidol,[17 40 53 75 84 85 88 99 111 147 175 176 312 317 368 415 419] behavior therapy,[19 94 95 163 379 375 493] psychotherapy, and manipulation of the environment.

In summary it would seem reasonable (1) to include all vocal tics (and not merely coprolalia) associated with multiple body tics under the heading of Gilles de la Tourette's syndrome, (2) to study the long-term prognosis of this condition by reviewing both published and previously unpublished cases, and, finally (3) to carry out a double-blind controlled trial of haloperidol in a larger series of cases than previously published.

Gilles de la Tourette's Syndrome. Volume 1: International Registry, p. 7-12, edited by F. Abuzzahab Sr. and F. Anderson. Mason Publishing Co., St. Paul ©1976.

GILLES DE LA TOURETTE'S SYNDROME A FOLLOW-UP OF FOUR CASES AND A NEW CASE REPORT

S.J.M. Fernando, M.A., M.B., B.Ch., D.P.M.

Consultant Psychiatrist,
Claybury Hospital
Woodford Bridge,
Essex, England

Six adults suffering from Gilles de la Tourette's syndrome have been reported by the author.[167, 168] Of these six, one died before her case was reported, and the man whose whereabouts were unknown in 1966[167] remains untraceable. The remaining four patients (three women and a man) have been followed up by means of correspondence with the patients and/or their general practitioners or personal interview of the patient. Brief follow-up reports are given here of the four previously reported cases together with a new case report.

CASE REPORTS

Case 1

This woman (M.P.) whose case was reported in 1967, is now aged 27½, single, and living with her parents. The patient reports that her recovery at about age 18 about nine years ago[167] has been maintained without any medication. She attributes her past illness to the disturbed childhood relationship with her father and the later mental strain of being "observed by people" — a reference to her frequent contact with doctors.

Case 2

This man (C.H.) originally reported in 1967 has been followed-up personally by the author at 6- to 12-month intervals. He is now aged 36, divorced from his wife on the grounds of her adultery, and courting a widow of about his own age. He continues to maintain a good work record. When started on haloperidol in July, 1966, he required a daily dose of 7.5 mg for maximal symptom control. Two months later he was able to reduce the daily dosage to 3 mg while maintaining the same degree of symptom control. When seen in May, 1970, he reported that his haloperidol requirement had been a mere 1.5 mg daily for nearly a year, but that omission of the drug had always resulted in a relapse of his condition within 2 or 3 days. While on haloperidol his motor tics are completely controlled, but barking noises with occasional muffled obscenities continue, although at a much lower frequency and intensity than in the past. Improvement has now been maintained for over 4½ years.

Case 3

This woman (C.S.), whose case was reported in 1968, is now a 25½-year-old married woman with two children. Although her tics had been sufficiently severe during her first pregnancy in 1965/6 and again about a year later in 1967 for her to seek psychiatric outpatient treatment,[168] her general practitioner reports that she carried a second pregnancy to term in 1968 with no ill effects. Her general practitioner does not consider that she shows any psychiatric symptoms or tics of any sort at present. The tentative conclusion to be drawn from her report and the meager hospital psychiatric outpatient notes on her case is that the patient suffered from tics of a varying intensity until May, 1967 (or later), but has been completely symptom-free since 1968, without receiving any medication. In view of her past difficulties and her possibly precarious adjustment, it seemed unwise to contact the patient directly for more conclusive information.

Case 4

This woman's (P.P.) case was originally reported in 1968. The patient is now a 29-year-old married woman with four children. The original history[168] reported that she had improved considerably without any medication between the ages of 19 and 26. Her general practitioner reports that further improvement has continued to occur. He observes that the patient is troubled now by a single tic of her neck — a solitary symptom, which itself is improving. He describes her as a "competent, hardworking and most charming" woman with "high standards and impeccable conduct."

Case 5

This new case is that of a married housewife (J.T.) aged 43½ who was referred to the author in December, 1968. She was the younger of two children and the only girl born to French parents living in Northern France. Her father being a violent man and a heavy drinker, her childhood was characterised by constant parental quarrelling. There is no family history of tics, but a maternal aunt was probably psychotic. Early development was normal until the onset of excessive blinking and grimacing at the age of 8-9. She had an average schooling between 6 and 14 years. She was unhappy in her first school because of an unnecessarily punitive teacher. She recalls being frequently reprimanded for restlessness and being locked in a dark cellar on one occasion for not learning a lesson. The tics began a few months before she was removed from her first school (at about the age of 9) because of her unhappiness there, and about that time she was frightened by being bitten by a dog. She was very happy at her next school, but the tics continued unabated, although she saw several doctors over the next 2 years.

She left school at 14 just before the outbreak of war in 1939 and stayed at home to help her mother, who was suffering from "dropsy." Jerks of her limbs began about one year later, and all her symptoms progressively worsened over the next 4 years. These years (1940-1944) were characterised for the patient by trials and tribulations of war as well as domestic stress in the form of parental dissension and the illness of her mother. The tics worsened at about the age of 18, particularly after she was assaulted by Nazi S.S. men in 1943-4. In 1944 her parents separated, and one year later her mother died. Soon afterwards, her future husband, whom she had met originally in 1940, renewed contact and in 1947 she came to England to join him. Unfortunately she was found to suffer from tuberculosis, requiring treatment. Muffled, cough-like vocalizations began in 1948 (about age 23), but these remained "slight" for nearly 5 years.

In 1952-3 (age 27) she began to utter nonspecific explosive noises. Vocal and motor tics worsened progressively over the next 15 years, resulting in a need to restrict her social life considerably. Her symptoms were unaffected by 3 pregnancies, although she noticed a two-month improvement after delivery of her first child in 1951. In 1949 she was treated with carbon dioxide inhalations without effect, and between 1962 and 1968 she took chlordiazepoxide with no benefit. In spite of her symptoms and consequent social difficulties, she has remained cheerful and friendly, although of a "nervous" disposition. She has never suffered from obsessional symptoms but is house-proud and fastidious about cleanliness. She is happily married with four children aged 17, 11, and twins of 7.

When seen at the clinic in 1968 she exhibited occasional blinking but no obvious grimacing. There were frequent jerking movements of all limbs which were sometimes co-ordinated into a "jump." The movements were usually accompanied by explosive, indistinct, complex noises which were sometimes almost recognizable to the author as a muted mixture of "bugger," and "Maman." (In fact, her husband claimed he heard "bugger," and the patient insisted it was "Maman.") Her husband reported that her tics were absent during sleep. They were reduced in intensity when she was relaxed (*e.g.*, sitting at home with her family), and exacerbated under social stress (*e.g.*, travelling in a bus, or shopping in a crowd). They were controllable voluntarily for 3 or 4 minutes with a subjective rise of tension and occasionally disappeared for up to 5 minutes at a time while her attention was absorbed in a television program or deep conversation with a friend. There was no evidence of echolalia or subjective awareness of a need to call out words.

She was diagnosed as suffering from Gilles de la Tourette's syndrome. There was no evidence of depression or other psychiatric illness. Her intelligence quotient on the Wechsler Adult Intelligence Scale (WAIS) was 92. Her response to the Rorshach was "controlled, defensive, and conventional." Electroencephalograpy showed mild, nonspecific abnormalities with no evidence of lateralization or localized abnormality.

Two sessions of direct suggestion under hypnosis produced no lasting effect, but all the tics were diminished in intensity and frequency during a light trance with complete relapse at its termination. Treatment with haloperidol, 4.5 mg daily, and orphenadrine hydrochloride, 150 mg daily, for one week produced no change. Within 48 hours of increasing the dosage of haloperidol to 7.5 mg daily a dramatic improvement occurred in all symptoms. However, on the seventh day on this dosage, having developed drowsiness, lethargy, dryness of mouth, difficulty in visual accommodation and tremor, the patient stopped her medication. She was persuaded to recommence haloperidol at the lower (originally ineffective) dosage (together with orphenadrine hydrochloride), increasing it by 1.5 mg (1 tablet) every 3 days to a level which was tolerable to her. She reported in a week that she was taking 6.0 mg of haloperidol together with 300 mg of orphenadrine hydrochloride daily. Symptoms were slightly controlled on this dosage and she agreed to continue the medication. One week later she developed a febrile illness with malaise, anorexia, and nausea. This was treated by her general practitioner as "glandular fever." The patient discontinued the haloperidol in case it interfered with the medication prescribed by her general practitioner. Six weeks later, full blood count, liver function, and Paul Bunnell tests were normal, but haloperidol was not recommended because the patient failed to keep her next appointment. Later, her husband wrote to the author that his wife was unwilling to continue treatment because she felt that the medication had "changed her personality to a point which frightened her," in spite of symptomatic improvement. Recent enquiry (July, 1970) revealed that her symptoms persist, and she continues to refuse treatment.

DISCUSSION

The four cases followed up and the new case reported serve to emphasize the complexity of the nature of this syndrome while supporting the value of haloperidol in controlling its symptoms. The efficacy of haloperidol in effecting a suppression of the tics of patients suffering from Gilles de la Tourette's syndrome and possible other diseases[99] is no longer in doubt, but the effects on the condition of long-term treatment with the drug are not known. Our case 2 (C.H.) has found that omission of haloperidol results in complete relapse, but, on the other hand, he has managed to reduce the dosage he needs to an almost minimal one. This may indicate an increasing sensitivity to the drug, or else since other factors aggravating his condition have eased up he has required less help from the drug in controlling his tics. From a personal knowledge of the patient's problems and reactions, the author tends to favor the latter explanation, but of course no conclusions can be drawn from such a subjective impression in one case. One must await follow-up reports of other patients suffering from this syndrome who have been on long-term haloperidol medication. Indeed, the author has recently met one such patient who developed a tolerance to the drug requiring a change to a similar drug (Fernando, in press).

A pleasing feature of the three women patients who were followed up (Cases 1, 3 and 4) is that all of them are now leading reasonably happy and normal lives with their respective families while receiving no medication. All these women had a classical history of the condition, resulting in a severe disruption of their adolescence and, in two cases, their childhood. One (Case 1) was given a poor prognosis and considered untreatable during her teens but recovered completely after leaving her parents and has showed no signs of relapse on returning to her parents. Her recent comments indicate that getting away from doctors may have been as therapeutic to her as leaving home. The other two women are functioning reasonably well as housewives and mothers, suffering from no particular psychiatric problems, although in one case (Case 3) the stability of the psychological improvement is in some doubt. It is remarkable that none of these three women received haloperidol.

The new case (Case 5) reported is unusual in that the diagnosis was not made until the patient was in her early forties, happily married with four children. The beneficial effect of haloperidol was expected, but the extent of the side effects was not. The refusal of the patient to continue treatment was puzzling both to the therapist and to the patient's husband. It may be argued that this was a result of poor management or mistrust of the therapist by the patient. However, the possibility must be faced that treatment with haloperidol did indeed result in a subtle and subjectively appreciated unwelcome "change of personality." Alternatively, one could speculate on the psychopathology of her utterances. Perhaps it is significant that "Maman" is what the woman claimed to shout, while "bugger" was what frequently emerged. Her refusal to continue treatment — which did undoubtedly suppress these explosive utterances — may be looked on as an indication of a subconscious psychological need to continue making these utterances. Perhaps when (or if) she no longer needs to do so, she would then come for treatment and allow haloperidol to suppress the utterances — or else emulate our other women patients reported in this paper and improve "spontaneously."

SUMMARY

Follow-up reports on four cases indicate that three (all women) have recovered or nearly recovered without medication. One man who improved on haloperidol continues to maintain his improvement having reduced the dosage of the drug over the years. A new case is reported of a woman who improved symptomatically on haloperidol but refused to continue treatment, claiming that the drug induced a "change of personality." The significance of some of the features of the cases reported are discussed. It is concluded that although haloperidol is of undoubted value, its effect appears to be symptom-suppression rather than curative; on the other hand, complete and sustained recovery is possible without medication.

Gilles de la Tourette's Syndrome. Volume 1: International Registry, p. 13-17, edited by F. Abuzzahab Sr. and F. Anderson. Mason Publishing Co., St. Paul ©1976.

FOLLOW-UP OF TIC SYNDROME

Alexander R. Lucas, M.D.
Adolescent Psychiatry Section
Mayo Clinic
Rochester, Minnesota 55901 U.S.A.

In 1967 we reported a clinical study of 15 children with tic syndrome (Gilles de la Tourette's disease) in which we reviewed histories, family dynamics, results of psychological evaluations, and academic performance.[286] The electroencephalograms have been described elsewhere.[287] In addition, we described the progression of the illness and reported follow-up status for periods varying from 2 to 15 years after patients were first seen. Several types of family interaction were discerned, with most of the children coming from families where there was severe and diffuse **expression** of aggression in home, or from families where there was excessive emphasis on the **inhibition** of both agression and negativism in the home. Approximately half of the children had psychological test findings and showed learning difficulties highly suggestive of encephalopathy. The others demonstrated no such deficits. The treatment plan was described, involving in most cases a combination of residential treatment, individual psychotherapy, and pharmacotherapy.

We have continued to see several of these children periodically, some in continuing therapy and others for follow-up. Their current status is now described, and five new cases are reported, making a total of 20 cases, 4 female and 16 male.

Two patients had previously been lost to follow-up and still have not been located. Those two (Cases 1 and 5) are now 32 and 26 years of age. The other 18 patients range in age from 14 to 29. Table 1 summarizes the 20 cases.

TABLE 1: SUMMARY OF TWENTY CASES OF TOURETTE'S SYNDROME

Case No.	Sex	Age in 1970	Age at onset	Age first seen	IQ	Encephalopathy and learning disabilities*	EEG	Family pattern +	Years of follow-up	Status of tic syndrome	Scholastic record	Social and personal adjustment
1	F	32	8-	11	118	C	Mildly abnormal	I	2	Improved	No difficulties	Good
2	F	29	8	10	107	C	—	II	15	Almost absent	Graduated from high school	Married, one child
3	M	27	4	10	104	B	Dysrhythmia gr. 1, gen.	II	13	Improved	Attended college	Fair
4	M	28	7	12	88	A	—	II	11	Improved	Graduated from university	Fair
5	M	26	6	11	146	C	—	I	5	Improved	Graduated from high school	Joined marine corps
6	M	21	5-	9	98	A	Dysrhythmia	II	12	Almost absent	Unable to complete high school	Repeated psych. hospitalizations
7	M	24	10	15	93	C	—	II	5	Almost absent	Attended college	Enlisted in army
8	M	24	9	15	102	B	—	I	5	Persisted	Quit school in 11th grade	Married, working with father

Case No.	Sex	Age in 1970	Age at onset	Age first seen	IQ	Enceph- alopathy and learning disabil- ities*	EEG	Family pattern+	Years of follow- up	Status of tic syndrome	Scholastic record	Social and personal adjustment
9	M	18	4	9	101	A	Dysrhythmia gr. 2, gen.	I	9	Absent	Quit school in 11th grade	Works as painter
10	M	19	6	11	114	B	Normal	II	5	Almost absent	Mild diffi- culties in high school	Good
11	M	18	8	11	90	A	Normal	II	7	Improved	Attends night school	Fair
12	F	15	6	9	91	A	Dysrhythmia gr. 2, gen.	I	6	Almost absent	Special education	Poor
13	M	14	6-	9	85	A	Normal	III	5	Improved	Special education	Poor
14	M	17	5	12	109	C	Normal	III	5	Improved	Graduating from high school	Good
15	F	17	5	11	108	C	Normal	II	6	Improved	Graduating from high school, will enter college	Fair
16	M	15	9	12	93	C	Dysrhythmia gr. 1, gen.	II	—			
17	M	23	7	13	98	B	Normal	I	9	Improved	Quit high school	Poor
18	M	16	8	14	62	A	Dysrhythmia gr. 3, gen.	II	—			
19	M	15	10	15	99	B	Dysrhythmia gr. 1, gen.	III	—			
20	M	18	14(?)	17	74	A	Normal	I	—			
	4 F 16 M	Range 14-32 years; X = 20.8	Range Ca. 4-14 years; X = Ca. 7¼	Range 9-17 years; X = 11.8	Range 62-146; S = 99.1	A = 8 cases B = 5 cases C = 7 cases	Data available on 15 cases, 7 of these show normal EEGs.	I = 7 cases II = 10 cases III = 3 cases	Range 2-15 years; X = 8	Data available on 16 cases: 1, tics absent; 5, tics almost absent; 9, improved; 1, tics persisted		

* As indicated by psychological test results and academic performance: **A** = definite signs of ençephalopathy and severe learning disabilities; **B** = questionable encephalopathy or moderately severe learning deficits; **C** = no signs of encephalopathy or learning deficits.

\+ **I** = severe and diffuse **expression of aggression in the home; II** = excessive emphasis on **inhibition** of agression and of negativism; **III** = no evidence of disturbance.

The writer's personal experience[285] during the past 12 years with tic syndrome patients suggests that typically the first signs of the disorder are seen between the ages of 4 and 10 and resemble the common transient tics of latency. Within several years, vocal noises develop which first resemble throat-clearing, coughs or grunts, and later, loud barking sounds.

Finally, usually near the time of puberty, coprolalia occurs. The progress of these symptoms occurs with unerring regularity, and on the basis of these symptoms, the diagnosis is made. Differential diagnosis was discussed in the 1967 paper. Schizophrenic children with bizarre, tic-like mannerisms and coprolalia were not included in the study.

Through adolescence the severity and frequency of the tics, both vocal and body tics, usually diminishes, and in early adulthood, the tics are generally much improved or almost absent. How much of this improvement is a reflection of treatment, and how much a reflection of the natural course of the disorder and maturation, is difficult to ascertain. On the basis of reported cases in whom severe tics have persisted long into adulthood, and the one case in our series in whom the tics persisted in severe form, but who left treatment after only two months of outpatient contacts, it would seem that treatment had an important influence on outcome. The nature of family dynamics and the presence or absence of encephalopathy appear to have no bearing on the outcome of the tics themselves. On the other hand, social and personality adjustment continued to be poor in a number of the patients during late adolescence and early adulthood. Those with signs of encephalopathy and severe learning deficits in childhood continued to have the greatest adjustment problems. Good intelligence, absence of signs of brain damage, and good academic performance were the best indicators of favorable eventual adjustment, regardless of the family dynamics.

On the basis of data which we still consider preliminary and incomplete, two early adult prototypes can tentatively be described:

1. The children who demonstrated signs of brain damage and severe learning deficits tend to become isolated, socially inept young adults prone to impulsive acts and frequent temper outbursts. While the tics have improved and may be almost absent, the life-long experience of social ostracism together with repeated failure and frustrations in school appear to have left permanent personality scars. Their job histories are erratic, with frequent job changes. They have difficulty persevering, react poorly to stress, and have difficulty accepting authority and supervision. In some instances, with unusually understanding and tolerant employers, they have been able to function effectively. An interesting finding is that two of the boys who had severe coordination deficits as young children have learned to play the piano with considerable competence. Another (Case 9) who was exceedingly clumsy as a child has become a skilled painter and decorator.

2. Those children who showed no signs of encephalopathy and who were academically competent were able to continue in school, graduate from high school, join the military service, or sometimes go on to college. They have better been able to compensate for their earlier frustrating experiences and have made an adequate social and personal adjustment. Still, interpersonal relationships have been difficult, although two have married. They have tended to be more introspective and to require more external support than the average individual.

Treatment needs to be multifaceted. Referral to a psychiatric facility usually occurs a few years after the onset of symptoms, when they have become severe enough to create major disruption in the home and at school. We have found a combination of residential treatment and psychotherapy necessary in most of our cases when symptoms had become so severe as to preclude regular school attendance. Medication is very helpful in the acute phase for most patients because it diminishes the severity of tics. Generally we have continued medication for several years, until late adolescence.

Follow-up of tic syndrome in our cases to date supports neither a psychotic nor a degenerative outcome in any of the cases. The tics almost invariably diminish in late adolescence, but social and personality adjustment is variable.

Gilles de la Tourette's Syndrome. Volume 1: International Registry, p. 19-24, edited by F. Abuzzahab Sr. and F. Anderson. Mason Publishing Co., St. Paul ©1976.

GILLES DE LA TOURETTE'S SYNDROME
A REPORT ON THREE CASES IN THE CHINESE

K. Singer, M.B., M.R.C.P.E., D.P.M.
Psychiatrist, Mental Health Service, Hong Kong
Head of Division of Psychiatry,
University of Hong Kong
Hong Kong Psychiatric Centre,
High Street, Hong Kong

The value of descriptive studies of psychiatric disorders in non-western cultures need not be emphasized. As regards Gilles de la Tourette's syndrome there was no report of its occurrence outside the Caucasian and Negro races and the Western culture till the author in 1963 described a case in a Chinese boy in Hong Kong.[426] Since then, isolated cases are said to have been seen in Taiwan (Hsu, personal communication, 1969), Korea (Lee, personal communication, 1970), and Thailand (Suwana, personal communication, 1970), and there have been reports of cases in India.[374 427]

The paucity of reports on this condition in non-Western cultures is accounted for not only by the lack of psychiatric facilities but also by the actual rarity of the condition. Estimates of the number of cases described in the literature range from 69[167] to 460 (Abuzzahab, personal communication, 1970), depending on the diagnostic criteria used. There is no controversy about the diagnosis of the full-blown syndrome, the features of which include multiple motor tics, vocal tics, coprolalia, and echophenomena such as echolalia and echopraxia. Onset in childhood and a prolonged and deteriorating course are regarded as typical and by some as essential for diagnosis. Only a handful of the reported cases fulfill all these criteria. In practice, diagnosis has been made on the basis of multiple tics and one or more of the other features, of which coprolalia is considered the most pathognomonic. Recently there has been a tendency to diagnose on a more liberal basis, multiple motor and vocal tics being thought sufficient.[101 374] Vocal tics would include not only loud, unprovoked utterances which are rare, bizarre, have a coprolalic quality and are considered typical of the syndrome, but also repetitive throat noises such as "grunting" and those involved in coughing and clearing of the throat. These noises are common and shade into those of the normal. Diagnosis on the basis of motor and vocal tics alone would therefore drain the syndrome of its rich and distinctive phenomenology and leave in its place a commonplace condition no more than a rather severe version of simple tics. Until we know more about the nosological position of Tourette's syndrome, it is probably wise to retain the stricter diagnostic criteria.

Because of the rarity of reports of the condition in non-Western cultures and outside the white and Negro races, it is felt that even isolated cases should not go unrecorded, especially when the etiology is largely unknown. Three cases are therefore described in this paper, two of them previously unreported, these being the only examples of the condition in the Chinese in the literature. They also show certain features not previously reported. Because of the necessity for follow-up studies which are lacking in most cases in the literature, this paper gives the follow-up on one case previously reported [426] and describes 2 new cases. All were seen in Hong Kong.

Case 1

This previously reported case[426] was that of a Chinese boy, 15 years old when first seen in 1960. The main features were onset at 8 of multiple tics followed by coprolalia and echolalia. Associated anxiety and obsessional phenomena were marked. Intelligence was above average and previous personality timid and obsessional. There was no evidence of organic lesion. He had no family history of tics or neuropsychiatric disorder. He made good improvement with a course of chlordiazepoxide (Librium) and isocarboxazid (Marplan). His tics became much diminished, and he had only very occasional coprolalia and echolalia. Eight months after withdrawal of medication, he maintained his improvement.

The patient was not seen again till December, 1969, which was for follow-up. He had received no treatment since 1962. Aged 24, he was a postman in a rural area, led a very quiet life, had no friends, and was regarded locally as an eccentric. His condition had fluctuated somewhat over the years, but on the whole he had maintained his improvement with respect to his tics, coprolalia, and echolalia. Anxiety and obsessional phenomena were somewhat worse.

Case 2

This 17-year-old Chinese male was first seen in 1965 when he complained of jerky movements affecting the face and limbs. At 11 he had had rheumatic fever with arthritis. During the illness he began grimacing and blinking. Similar involuntary movements spread to the neck and limbs. Later he developed coughing and loud inarticulate noises (''hem,'' ''haa''). At 12 his utterances took on an obscene character (''tiu,'' which is Chinese for ''fuck''). These were made several times daily but were usually controllable in the presence of others. His symptoms appeared closely related to ordinary daily stresses and over the years fluctuated considerably. At 21, inability to resist carrying on long monologues with himself became the chief complaint. They consisted of reminiscences, criticisms, and comments on recent activity and events, intermixed with utterances like ''Shut up!'', ''Behave properly.'' ''Why are you such a nuisance?'' addressed to himself in an effort, he said, to control his symptoms. He would talk loudly thus when alone, but also in a lower voice in the presence of others, much to his own embarrassment. He felt compelled to name and describe objects immediately as he saw them. He would also describe people's actions, *e.g.*, the examiner jotting down notes. Occasionally he could not resist repeating immediately and seemingly without purpose what others said. For example, on hearing the remark, ''You are just too awful,'' in a dialogue between two others, he had to repeat this to himself. He also had a tendency to repeat his own words, *e.g.*, ''Now this is difficult, this is difficult.'' These phenomena occurred several times daily. Tension, irritability, and ruminations were prominent. Other features were mild depression, insomnia, and impairment of concentration. His intelligence was average and his previous personality markedly obsessional.

Birth and development were normal. He was 9th of 12 children in a family of the lower-income group and had 6 years' schooling. Family history was negative for tics and neuropsychiatric disorder. Making ends meet was a constant family preoccupation. He had difficulty in holding his job as a warden in a penitentiary chiefly because of his colleagues' ridicule.

Physically he had well-compensated chronic rheumatic heart disease with mitral and aortic valvular involvement. Routine laboratory investigations were negative.

He was treated with diazepam (Valium), chlordiazepoxide (Librium), isocarboxazid (Marplan), and haloperidol (Haldol) at different times. He did best when maintained on haloperidol, 0.5 mgm t.i.d. achieving moderate improvement in all his symptoms.

In summary, the main features were a boyhood onset of a progressive disorder with multiple tics, vocal tics, coprolalia, echolalia, pallilalia, compulsive monologizing, and anxiety and obsessional phenomena. Previous personality was markedly obsessional.

Case 3

This Chinese man, who was 38 years old, when he first presented himself in 1968, complained chiefly of being unable to resist carrying on a monologue with himself and to a lesser extent of feeling compelled to repeat other people's words immediately on hearing them.

At 10 he began having tics involving the face — blinking, mouth twisting, raising eyebrows. They were infrequent and not the subject of complaint. His personality was obsessional and hypothymic, and he suffered chronically from a mild to moderate nervousness. Nevertheless he was able to become an architect and to work (admittedly with considerable support) in his father's firm. At 32 he took a turn for the worse, suffering several bouts of panic for no apparent reason. Thereafter his nervousness became marked. It was at this time that he began to conduct monologues with himself. The content referred chiefly to daily happenings. He also felt compelled to repeat words immediately on hearing them. For example, on one occasion he repeated "Provision Merchange" 6-7 times. This symptom impaired his powers of comprehension. He found himself unable to follow the dialogue in a movie because he had to repeat it to himself. He also felt compelled to imitate the simple gestures of the characters. This compulsion to imitate also extended, though to a lesser extent, to the live situation. Thus, when the examiner picked up a telephone, the patient had great difficulty in restraining himself from doing the same, as he afterwards related. If confronted with an open book, he was unable to resist reading aloud. Occasionally he made loud, abrupt, inarticulate cries which sometimes took on an obscene character ("tiu") but this was only when he was alone. Obsessional and depressive features were prominent.

His electroencephalogram showed occasional theta waves in the frontal regions. Otherwise physical and laboratory investigations were negative.

Birth and milestones of development were normal. He was the eldest of 6 children. Four siblings had history of "nervous breakdowns" associated with sitting for examinations. His mother was very highly strung. He was single and lived with his mother and siblings. The family atmosphere was strained. His father lived apart with a concubine, and the patient was obviously over-dependent on, and probably had suppressed hostility for, him.

He was treated with amitryptyline, chlordiazepoxide, diazepam, isocarboxazid, amobarbitol, and haloperidol in various combinations. Haloperidol had a selective effect on tics, diazepam on tension. The value of the other drugs was not evident.

In summary, the main features were multiple tics, compulsive monologizing, echolalia, pallilalia, coprolalia, anxiety, and obsessional phenomena.

COMMENT

The major point of interest in these three cases is their occurrence in the Chinese. Taking also into account the isolated reports of the occurrence of Tourette's syndrome in various other orientals, it now seems reasonable to conclude what was previously assumed without adequate basis: That the condition is worldwide and found in all races and cultures. Its occurrence in all cultures differentiates it from latah, with which the condition has been confused by some. Latah is confined to certain "primitive" cultures, and this is one of several points of difference between the two conditions.

As regards clinical features, all 3 cases were typical: Affecting males, having onset in childhood (although in Case 3 there was a wide time gap between onset of tics and the other features), and being characterized by multiple tics, coprolalia, and echo-phenomena. However, features shown by these cases not reported previously so far as I can trace were compulsive talking to oneself or compulsive monologizing (prominent in Case 2 and 3), compulsive reflex-like naming of objects and description of actions as they were perceived (Case 2), and compulsive reading aloud (Case 3). These features may be regarded as congruent with the rest of the syndrome and as examples of echo-phenomena. Thus, compulsive naming of objects would be echoing in verbal form of objects perceived; compulsive description of actions, echoing in verbal form of actions perceived; compulsive reading aloud, echoing in verbal form of written words perceived; and compulsive monologizing, similar to echoing of mental imagery.

Relevant to etiology is the marked obsessional coloring found in these cases, both in respect of the illness and of the previous personality. The condition could indeed be clinically regarded as a form of obsessional neurosis with predominantly motor phenomena of a specific kind. However, although certain authors have regarded the condition as obsessional in nature, there is controversy about this, and certainly obsessional features have been lacking in some reported cases.

As regards the course and prognosis, the length of illness in these cases ranged from 13 to 34 years. Throughout the illness, the condition fluctuated with stresses, but none showed any tendency towards deterioration or psychosis, and this is in agreement with recent findings.[46] It is also noteworthy that 2 of the cases improved moderately with haloperidol.

Concerning psychodynamics, abnormal family patterns and in particular suppressed hostility to parent figures could be discerned in all. These are, however, inferences within a theoretical framework rather than objective data and are of limited value for comparative purposes.

As regards organic pathology, an association with chorea has often been reported in the literature — in 14 out of 69 cases in one review — but in none of these was actual evidence of rheumatic pathology found.[167] In the present series, one patient had a proven rheumatic pathology, and the illness started when he had rheumatic fever at 11.

Finally, it is of interest that the coprolalic utterances in Chinese were of the same literal meaning as those of English-speaking patients. This is not surprising as the Chinese attitude to sex, with respect to equating it with the shameful and dirty, is similar to that in the West. It might prove fruitful to study the utterances in cultures with different attitudes to see what part culture plays in these utterances.[156]

SUMMARY

Three cases of Gilles de la Tourette's syndrome are described, these apparently being the only examples in the Chinese so far reported in the literature. Apart from the usual features of the condition — multiple tics, coprolalia, echolalia and echopraxia — some of the cases also showed features not previously described. These were compulsive monologizing, compulsive reflex-like naming of objects and description of actions perceived, and compulsive reading aloud. It is surmised that these are examples of echo-phenomena and congruent with the rest of the syndrome.

Brief mention is made of the occurrence of this condition in various cultures. It seems reasonable to conclude that the condition is worldwide and found in all cultures and races.

Gilles de la Tourette's Syndrome. Volume 1: International Registry, p. 25-32, edited by F. Abuzzahab Sr. and F. Anderson. Mason Publishing Co., St. Paul ©1976.

THE NATURE OF TICS AND GILLES DE LA TOURETTE'S SYNDROME

J. A. Corbett, M.R.C.P., D.C.H., D.P.M.
Maudsley Hospital,
Denmark Hill
London S.E. 5 England

Gilles de la Tourette[198] quoted a statement made by Bouteille in 1818 referring to chorea: "Everything is extraordinary in this disease; the name is ridiculous, its symptoms peculiar, its character equivocal, its cause unknown and the treatment problematical." Although Itard[532] in 1825 had described a case of a 26-year-old woman who, at the age of seven, began to have jerking tics of the arms spreading to other parts of her body with eventual vocalizations and obscene epithets, Tourette's name is usually given to the syndrome he described in 1885 in which tics of the face or upper limbs spread to the rest of the body to be followed by inarticulate sounds and coprolalia, a condition which bears some resemblance to his quotation, given above.

Of the eight cases Tourette described, only five progressed to coprolalia, and of over a hundred appearing in the literature since Tourette's description, nearly half had vocal tics but not coprolalia.[243 167]

Although Tourette's syndrome is rare, tics are very frequent in childhood, and various writers have estimated that they occur at some time in between 4 and 23% of 5-year-old children,[51 290 377] although less frequently in 10 and 11-year-olds.[399] These tics are often transient, most usually involving eye blinking, with a descending order of frequency down the rest of the face and body, but they tend to be more persistent if peripheral parts of the body are involved.[101 316 485] The description of Kanner[241] of "quick, sudden and frequently repeated movements of circumscribed groups of muscles, serving no apparent purpose," is perhaps most fitting for this type of tic.

These tics tend to be more persistent in adolescence when they come to be associated with vocalizations, coprolalia, echopraxia, and copropraxia but, even then, the outlook is not as poor as Tourette himself suggested. Over 60% recover from their tics and are no longer handicapped by them in adult life, although there is a tendency for the psychiatric symptoms with which they are commonly associated, particularly anxiety[101 457] to persist.

In considering the nature of these symptoms, it is important to decide whether simple or multiple tics and the fully developed Gilles de la Tourette's syndrome are distinct conditions, as is frequently emphasized in the literature, or rather different stages in the development of one syndrome, the fully fledged form of which is distinguished by vocalizations and coprolalia.

In order to examine this further, the anamnestic data of three groups of patients has been examined. Group A comprised 171 previously described[101] children and adults attending Maudsley Hospital and Brixton Child Guidance Unit between 1948 and 1965. Of these patients 23% suffered from vocal tics in association with tics of other parts of the body and might thus be described as cases of Gilles de la Tourette's syndrome, but the remainder, who comprised the majority of cases, had simple or multiple body tics.

Group B comprised 31 patients with vocal and multiple body tics, and Group C, 20 patients with coprolalia and multiple body tics. Some of these

TABLE I

Comparative Data on the Three Groups of Patients

	Male: Female Ratio	Mean age of			In-patient %	Abnormal EEG	Mean I.Q.			Distribution of tics, %					Prognosis		
		Tic Onset	First Exam	Coprolalia Onset			Full-Scale	Verbal	Performance	Vocal	Eyes	Face, Head, and Neck	Upper Limbs	Lower Limbs	Improved %	No Change %	Worse %
Group A (N = 171) Vocal tics + body tics (23%) Simple or multiple body tics (77%)	3.6:1	7.3	10.2	—	0	0	94	?	?	23	82	58	17	10	94	6	0
Group B (N = 31) Vocal + multiple body tics	3.5:1	7.9	14.1	12.0	6.7	8/15 (53%)	99	95	90	100	70	70	28	20	66	28	6
Group C (N = 20) Coprolalia + multiple body tics	6.5:1	8.9	15.0	13.8	4.1	5/13 (38%)	95	102	106	80	80	65	60	50	55	30	15

were included in the original study while others have been seen since. Patients with isolated vocal tics or coprolalia were excluded.

There was a higher proportion of boys with coprolalia and a tendency for those with vocal tics and coprolalia to attend for treatment later in adolescence. The age of onset of both tics and vocalizations was also slightly higher in the cases of Gilles de la Tourette's syndrome. With the exception of the sex difference, which will be discussed later, all these differences can easily be explained by the development of coprolalia as a later feature in the condition, while the tendency for more patients with coprolalia to be admitted as inpatients is, presumably, due to the embarrassing nature of the symptom and the increased severity of the psychiatric concomitants.

TABLE II

Psychiatric Symptoms and Family History Data

		Percent of patients in each group showing		
		A	**B**	**C**
I.	Psychiatric Symptoms in Patient			
	Antisocial			
	Aggression	37	29	40
	Destructive	30	10	10
	Lying	21	3	10
	Disobedient	—	23	30
	Stealing	17	13	10
	Truanting	17	13	10
	Neurotic			
	Anxiety	34	27	20
	Depression	8	13	10
	Obsessional	12	3	10
II.	Family History Data			
	Sociopathic factors in family	—	13	40
	Parental psychiatric illness	31	28	55
	Tics in parents and sibs	—	10	15
	Chorea in parents or sibs	—	10	5

Psychiatric symptoms, in addition to the tics, were found in the vast majority of cases in all three groups, although there may have been some bias due to the fact that the patients were attending psychiatric clinics. The only difference with cases of Tourette's syndrome was the increased severity of the same symptoms.

Electroencephalograms were not done in all cases, but abnormal EEGs were found more frequently in Group B. However, there was no evidence that the frequency of brain damage, assessed clinically, was significantly different in the three groups, and the IQ results were similar in all three. The failure to find a higher verbal versus performance discrepancy in Group C perhaps supports the suggestion that brain damage was not a distinguishing feature.

Sociopathic factors in the family, parental psychiatric illness (most usually affective illness in mothers) and a family history of tics or chorea were frequent in all three groups, and several times the frequency in the general patient population attending the hospital.[101] It was, however, greatest in those patients with coprolalia.

There was a tendency for both vocal tics and coprolalia to be associated with multiple body tics, but, in those patients with coprolalia, other tics tended to be more widely distributed and severe. The prognosis in all three groups was similar. Thus, apart from a tendency for patients with Gilles de la Tourette's syndrome to be more severely affected later in adolescence and to be characterized by vocal tics and coprolalia, this data fails to show any fundamental difference from children with simple tics. This is borne out by the response of the symptoms to treatment with haloperidol[99 103 307] with behavior therapy[19 94 147 238 379 457 493] and psychotherapy.[264 495]

It is thus perhaps relevant to discuss the possible nature of these symptoms together. At the time that Tourette gave his original description, papers were published on latah,[347] myriachit[213] and the "Jumping" Frenchmen of Maine[24] and Tourette identified the condition with these reactions. Latah is found among the Malays and consists of a severe startle reaction, echopraxia, echolalia, automatic obedience, and coprolalia. Myriachit is a similar condition, one of a group classified as "Arctic Hysteria,"[2 492] while the Jumpers of Maine display similar features as part of a religious ritual. Yap suggests that latah and similar reactions are traumatic or fear neuroses found in primitive cultures — cultures with limited control over the environment. They differ from Tourette's syndrome in being culture-bound, (in that the startle response is always prompted by some external stimulus), in being more frequent in females, and in the fact that coprolalia is invariably present.

Most recent writers have dismissed the notion of any connection between the two phenomena, but, although clearly distinct conditions, the underlying pathology may not be entirely dissimilar. Ferenczi[165] quotes a discussion with Freud about the meaning and significance of tics in which Freud suggested that "there was an organic factor in the question."

Organic factors have long been suggested as of underlying importance and at least five different groups of theories have been put forward:

1. Tics are initiated by local irritation (*e.g.*, infection of the upper respiratory tract).[61 68 416]

2. They are related to movement restraint in early infancy.[277]
3. Generalized brain damage underlies them.[359]
4. There is a focal neurological lesion.[97]
5. They are related to chorea or epidemic encephalitis.[112]

Although tics occur at an age when upper respiratory infections are common in the Maudsley series there was no evidence that this was a major contributory factor or that movement restraint, which may be responsible for the tic-like movements of battery hens or horses, is important in children, confirming the findings of Bergmann who studied abnormal movements in children in an orthopaedic ward. While brain damage may be an important feature in some cases, most of the EEG abnormalities which are found are of a non-specific nature, and Pasamanick's finding[359] of an increased number of reproductive casualties in a group of tiqueurs is based on a very small series and was not supported by the Maudsley data.

The suggestion of a lesion in the basal ganglia, while possible, is based on a positive autopsy finding of an immature cell structure of the corpus striatum in only one case of Gilles de la Tourette's syndrome[97] the similarity between tic movements and those following epidemic encephalitis[485] and the finding of an increased incidence of previous chorea in patients with tics.[112]

Difficulties in differential diagnosis may have contributed to this last observation, and we failed to confirm this finding in the more recent cases admittedly at a time when Sydenham's chorea was less frequent. A more recent piece of evidence supporting a more specific site of origin for tics has been the finding of a response to haloperidol of both tics and Gilles de la Tourette's syndrome.[99, 307]

An emotional cause for these symptoms is supported by theories ranging from that of the early psychoanalytic writers who saw the tics as symbolic of repressed desires (for example, hand-jerking tics as repressed impulses to masturbate),[164] or eye-blinking as crying corresponding to "fixation of the traumatic primal scene"[260] to the commonly observed finding of an increase in psychiatric disturbance among patients with both tics and Tourette's syndrome and also in their families.[99, 457] There was no definite tendency for tics to be associated with one particular symptom or psychiatric syndrome, although developmental disorders such as thumb-sucking, speech disorders, and encopresis, and obsessional and hypochondriacal disorders occurred significantly more frequently in patients with tics than in the general population of disturbed children attending the hospital. Tempers, aggression, truanting, and depression occurred significantly less frequently, although they were somewhat more marked in the cases of Gilles de la Tourette's syndrome who were hospitalized. This suggests that tiqueurs are not characterized by the overt expression of affect, and that the tics may be an alternative mode of affective response. Although obsessional symptoms were somewhat more common, they were not invariable, as suggested by Meige.[316]

From a therapeutic point of view, the contribution of the learning theorists to the etiology of tics has been most striking. Yates[493] saw tics as conditioned avoidance responses, evoked initially by stress and reinforced by reduction in anxiety. He and other workers followed the lead of Dunlap[149] in the successful treatment of tics by massed practice[238 379 475 493] and by operant methods.[19] This has even been extended to the treatment of Tourette's syndrome.[94] Learning theorists do not, however, discuss the nature of the initial avoidance response or the etiology of the associated psychiatric symptoms.

A striking similarity was found between both the distribution and nature of the movements in the tic syndrome and in the startle response, both when the frequency of the individual symptoms in the Maudsley series is considered, and when the movements are compared by high speed cinephotography.

TABLE III

Distribution of Movements in the Tic Syndrome and Startle Response*

	No. of Subjects			
	A	B	C	Startle Response
	185	31	20	32
Movements				
Eyes (blinking)	82%	70%	80%	86%
Face, head, and neck (flaring of nostril, baring of teeth, shrugging of shoulders, etc.)	58%	70%	65%	85%
Upper limbs (abduction of upper arms, flexion of elbows and fingers)	17%	28%	60%	25%
Lower limbs (extension of hips, flexion of knees)	10%	20%	50%	43%

* From Landis and Hunt [265]

The startle response was described in detail by Landis and Hunt.[265] One of the most interesting properties of this almost universal motor response to a sudden, powerful stimulis, (*e.g.*, a revolver shot) is that it can be conditioned using repeated paired presentation with a conditioned stimulus, (*e.g.*, a buzzer or light) and it then shows all the characteristics of a conditioned reflex providing a link with the learning theory of tics.

The concept of tics as a developmental disorder would fit in with this and is suggested by the sex ratio with an increased frequency in boys, restricted range and early age of onset, the tendency to remit after adolescence, and also by the association with other developmental disorders.[104]

The fact that tics both cause anxiety and improve following a reduction in anxiety, which may be reinforcing, accounts for the association with other psychiatric symptoms, while the greatly increased frequency in psychiatric illness in the parents of tiqueurs and adverse sociofamilial circumstances may provide both an anxiety-provoking environment for tiqueurs and contribute to their constitutional predisposition to emotional disturbance.

We are left with the interesting development of coprolalia in Tourette's syndrome. The fact that this is even more frequent in boys may be linked with their greater difficulty in the problem of control of aggression in adolescence. As MacDonald[289] has put it, "Tics occur at a time of life when the child is struggling with the problem of control." Following the use of CO_2 inhalation in a case of Tourette's syndrome by Michael,[322] MacDonald treated a girl with this condition by controlled abreaction using CO_2, pentothal, and amphetamine.

The coprolalic utterances, which are usually monosyllabic, may perhaps be accounted for by considering the ways in which the tiqueurs' perception and response to the tics serve to shape the form of the tics themselves. A specific formulation of such a "feedback" hypothesis was proposed by MacDonald. The recent description of Tourette's syndrome in different cultures in which the coprolalic utterances are determined more by their sexual content than by the sound of the words would support this hypothesis.[83 426 198] Perhaps the coprolalic patient is attempting unsuccessfully to carry out his own psychotherapy by verbalizing rather than acting out aggressive impulses as part of a disturbance of ego development.

Gilles de la Tourette's Syndrome. Volume 1: International Registry, p. 33-41, edited by F. Abuzzahab Sr. and F. Anderson. Mason Publishing Co., St. Paul ©1976.

GILLES DE LA TOURETTE'S SYNDROME: ITS COMPLICATION BY ALLERGY AND A RARE SYMPTOM

F. S. Abuzzahab Sr., M.D., Ph.D.
Clinical Associate Professor
Departments of Psychiatry, Pharmacology
and Family Practice and Community Health
University of Minnesota
Minneapolis, Minnesota 55455 U.S.A.

and

Floyd O. Anderson, M.D.
Resident in Psychiatry
University of Minnesota
Minneapolis, Minnesota 55455 U.S.A.

Gilles de la Tourette's syndrome is an esoteric disorder which has fascinated and frustrated medical professionals for decades. As is true with any malady with an obscure etiology, the medical literature abounds with hypotheses and speculation about its cause or causes.[5 18 162 172] Since the best source of clues in this search is obtained from case histories, it is essential to continue reporting diagnosed cases of the disorder until a definitive etiology and effective treatment are established.

Towards this end, we have published case reports of seven patients with Gilles de la Tourette's syndrome.[4] Recently, we have had the opportunity to treat four more patients suffering from this disorder, and include, with these four new case reports, extended follow-up information on the previously reported seven.

CASE REPORTS

Case 8

R.T., a 21-year-old white male, was admitted to Mayo Clinic in Rochester, Minnesota, in October of 1969 "to find better control or possible cure of Tourette's syndrome." Pregnancy, birth, and developmental milestones were all normal.

At the age of 4 he began suffering from involuntary movements in the face, flinging of an arm, and occasional jerks of the legs. By the age of 10 these paroxysmal tics were associated with a snorting or grunting sound. A dramatic increase in the frequency and severity of the paroxysms occurred in the spring of 1967, and subsequent to this, a seasonal variation became apparent, with exacerbation between May and September and relative remission during the colder months. In 1969, coprolalia was evident, with explosive utterances of monosyllabic sex words.

The tics and vocalizations in this patient are susceptible to brief voluntary postponement, and there is amelioration during sleep. Also, another typical pattern is present, that of relative refractory periods following each paroxysm.

The patient's mother reports a medical history that is all too common with this syndrome: "We originally went to a pediatrician, who told us he would outgrow the 'tics' and that we should 'relax, not pressure him, not talk about it to him.' Then, as time passed, with his condition steadily worsening, we took him to a general practitioner, a psychologist, a neurologist, three different psychiatrists, and a psychiatrist specializing in hypnosis. Finally, when he was 16 (1966) we read a newspaper article which discussed Gilles de la Tourette's syndrome. It described our son almost to a 'T.' We told his psychiatrist about it, but he dismissed it by saying that this condition is so rare that R. couldn't possibly have it."

In 1967 (age 17) his condition worsened, and a psychiatric consultation produced a diagnosis of Gilles de la Tourette's syndrome. Haloperidol was prescribed, but it did not give complete relief. The patient was maintained on 3 mg of haloperidol daily until his admission to Mayo Clinic. The neurologic examination revealed nothing in addition to the Tourette's syndrome save a dull ache behind the right eye and in the right half of his head, which was minor and readily responsive to aspirin. The physical examination revealed obesity and an easy fatigability secondary to it. X-ray and lab studies were within normal limits, and an electroencephalogram was also normal. No other psychometric results are available.

Various dosages of haloperidol were tried, with the best if not complete relief obtainable at an orthodox dose. The patient was discharged on a regimen of 3 mg haloperidol daily with ½ mg benztropine mesylate (Cogentin).

The unusual seasonal character of motor and vocal manifestations of the syndrome in this patient prompted his parents to consult an allergist. Sensitivity studies were conducted, revealing sensitivity to many allergens. A regimen of desensitization injections during the winter of 1969-70 produced a marked diminution of symptoms, and the administration of brompheniramine maleate (Dimetane) capsules in a dose of 20 mg every 8 hours produced nearly complete control through the summer of 1970, the time at which his symptoms were usually the worst. At one time he missed 3 consecutive injections with return of symptoms.

Case 9

C.C. is a seven-year-old girl whose difficulties started in May, 1970, at the age of six. The first symptoms noticed by her mother included frequent raising of the eyelids and "making big eyes." Subsequently she started sticking her tongue out of her mouth like a snake, followed by facial grimacing and nasal sniffing. The patient was first seen in late July, 1970.

There has been no report of coprolalia. Occasionally she says the words "damn it," but apparently not during the motor paroxysms described above. Her tics are absent during sleep and are more prevalent when she is excited. Past medical history reveals that the patient had bronchitis and received antibiotics three weeks before her tics began.

There is considerable friction between the mother and father of long duration. The father is domineering, rigid, and lacks understanding. "He gives C. too many spankings. He is always against us." The mother is still dependent on her own mother for support. She is nervous and has been taking medication.

The patient is an only child. Placenta previa at 34 weeks necessitated many transfusions, and at delivery she weighed only 4½ lbs and spent 5 weeks in an incubator. Normal milestones were reached, and she has finished first grade with exceptional reading ability. She has suffered from enuresis since May, 1970, the same time as her symptoms began.

During the psychiatric interview, the child was very hyperactive. In fact, she could not sit still. She elected to sit on the desk chair, which has wheels, and she was constantly moving the chair back and forth or swiveling. To decrease the grimaces of her mouth, she was chewing gum. Occasionally during the grimace, she would open her mouth as if blowing bubbles, thus deceiving the examiner as to whether this was an uncontrolled grimace or not. Nasal sniffing accompanied the grimace, and occasionally she would raise her eyelids. On the whole, however, she was a very pleasant, attractive child.

Hydroxyzine (Vistaril) and belladonna alkaloids and phenobarbital (Donnatal) were tried prior to haloperidol (Haldol), but these produced nightmares and drowsiness. Haloperidol was prescribed, 1 mg daily at that time, to be increased to 2 mg daily if needed.

One week later the tics (except for the sniffing) were under complete control. She was much calmer, and her hyperactivity was gone. Her mother and grandmother feel as if she is a new person. Her dose of haloperidol was raised to 2 mg daily in an attempt to eliminate the sniffing.

A follow-up interview in September, 1970, showed that she was doing well except for occasional sniffing, especially when she is excited. Her only complaints are tiredness and mild weight gain. The father was given a prescription for perphenazine (Trilafon), 2 mg t.i.d., for nervousness with no effect, while the mother claims to be calmer on doxepin HC1 (Sinequan).

The patient was seen in late October, November, and lastly December for progress reports. By December her tics were gone completely, and she was making adequate progress in school. Her medication remains haloperidol, 2 mg daily, which she takes at 4 p.m. to avoid tiredness during school. Although she is on the chubby side (65 lbs or 29.5 kg) her weight has somewhat stabilized.

Case 10

B.P., a 10-year-old white male, was admitted to the University of Minnesota Hospitals in June, 1970. He had developed a mild facial grimace at the age of 5, for which his parents scolded him, blaming it on too much T.V. There was no historical evidence of any precipitating event. During his eighth year he developed a vocal inarticulation described by the patient as a "frog sound." Later development of echolalia, coprolalia, echopraxia, and copropraxia prompted his referral to University Hospitals.

The patient presented with tics involving all facial mimic muscles, arms, and the right leg. The typical paroxysm involved a grimace, lashing arms, a foot stomp, and a guttural inarticulation. The patient related that he mimics words and gestures, swears, and makes obscene signs with his fingers. Echopraxia could readily be demonstrated in the interview, although echolalia and the coprophenomena were not overt. The symptoms appeared to be more apparent in his mother's presence.

Gestation, delivery, and developmental milestones were normal. The patient is the second of three children, and the family nervous history reveals a paternal uncle with tic douloureux, and three cousins with histories of seizures.

Intrafamily relations are strained. The patient, according to the father, is at constant war with his mother and has been since the onset of the syndrome. The mother is described as highstrung, and both parents have sought counseling with a psychologist.

The patient does average work in school, and presents as a well-nourished, cheerful boy. Physical examination was within normal limits, an EEG was normal, and the IQ is over 120.

Haloperidol was administered, initially 2.4 mg daily and finally 1.5 mg three times daily, and good control was achieved. It was necessary to administer 25 mg of diphenhydramine HC1 (Benadryl) twice daily to alleviate stiffness and fatigue. The patient was discharged two weeks after admission.

A follow-up interview in August, 1970, revealed a weight gain and persistent mild echophenomena, although good control of tics was maintained. His medications were not changed despite the complaint of tiredness and lethargy, although it was suggested that the haloperidol be administered at bedtime in an attempt to minimize the side effects of the drug.

The patient was readmitted to University Hospitals in February, 1971, when a head jerk proved refractory to diphenhydramine. Further weight gain led to the hypothesis that the haloperidol dosage was no longer adequate, and an increase to 2.5 mg three times daily proved effective. Benztropine mesylate (Cogentin) was prescribed, 1 mg daily.

Case 11

J.P., born May 4, 1955, was first seen at a St. Paul, Minnesota, clinic at the age of 7. He presented with multiple tics consisting of eye blinking, tics of the trunk and upper extremity, and guttural sounds described as "snorting." Psychological testing at the time revealed an IQ of 115 and indicated that the boy was considerably anxious about interpersonal relationships and appeared to have a great deal of "inhibited hostility and fearfulness." At this time it was also noted that the boy's parents were somewhat submissive and inhibited. Communication between family members was markedly restricted, and anger particularly seemed not permissible. A history of treatment at this time was not obtainable, except that there was no progress with the patient or his parents.

From 1963 to 1966 (ages 8-11), poor adjustment and performance in school led to extensive psychological testing with no diagnosis or effective treatments. IQ scores varied from 93 to 106, and motor symptoms slowly progressed. Regression, compulsivity, and depression were words frequently found in psychologists' reports.

The boy was first hospitalized in December, 1970, at a St. Paul, Minnesota, hospital. Besides a considerable array of tics and vocalizations, general tension and nervousness were noted. Coprolalia was absent. Some of the tests administered at this time were: (1) Wechsler Intelligence Scale for Children (WISC), (2) Bender-Gestalt, (3) Rorschach, (4) Thematic Apperception Test (TAT), (5) sentence completion, and (6) figure drawings.

No organic involvement was demonstrated, and full-scale WISC IQ was 93, with verbal IQ 100 and performance IQ 87. Projective tests clearly revealed psychological conflict, especially with his father. Strong aggressive feelings were found, but no psychoses were indicated. The diagnosis at that time was hysterical neurosis, with multiple tics, anxiety, and tension. Physical examination and lab tests were normal, and 4 mg of haloperidol per day was prescribed along with benztropine mesylate (Cogentin). The side effect of fatigue, in particular, led to the discontinuation of the medication, although slight improvement was noted.

We first saw the patient when he was admitted to Hastings State Hospital in Minnesota in March, 1971, with the same chief complaints as aforementioned. Interestingly, only now was a history of coprolalia obtained, common expressions of which were "goddamn it," "son of a bitch," and "fucker." The patient stated that he possibly picked up the tic from a neighbor boy who had tics. The boy's school progress remained poor.

The previous medical history revealed an apparently uncomplicated bout of measles at age 7, and fractures of the left ankle twice and clavicle once. In 1967 (age 12) he underwent an operation to insert a plastic disc in his left eye. His birth history includes a 72-hour labor with forceps delivery, but normal developmental milestones were achieved thereafter.

A family history of nervous disorders is not present. The patient has one sister, 20 years old. Family environment is still undesirable. The patient reports that his tics "make his father nervous," and that his parents fight "only when I am around." He also relates discord between himself and his sister. During the interview the patient expressed some thoughts of suicide, and said that he would use his haloperidol to overdose. He also appeared depressed, especially when discussing his family.

The diagnosis of Gilles de la Tourette's syndrome was made, and therapy consisted of haloperidol and amantadine HC1 (Symmetrel). Drowsiness and insignificant improvement of symptoms led to discontinuation of medication shortly thereafter. Currently, the patient shows no improvement, and schoolwork continues to be poor. He remains at Hastings State Hospital.

DISCUSSION

A possible clue to the mysteries of Gilles de la Tourette's syndrome is found in Case 8. There are no other reports in our master bibliography, containing close to 500 case histories, which involve the interaction of an acute allergic condition with this syndrome. The dramatic reversal in the severity of involvement upon treatment with desensitization therapy and antihistamines could imply that blood histamine levels affect the severity of symptoms. In support of this statement is the fact that a common feature of many Tourette's cases is the exacerbation of symptoms during an acute infectious process.

It is difficult, however, to pinpoint a mechanism for his histaminergic phenomenon. Histamine does not cross the blood-brain barrier, and, in the brain, it is a neurohumoral agent not located in mast cells. In an impressive review, Monnier *et al* [330] discuss the effects of histamine on the central nervous system. The only effect they found upon parenteral injection of histamine was a definite waking effect, as evidenced by decreased delta activity accompanied by increased reticulocortical, interlaminary thalamocortical, and hippocampocortical evoked potentials. This arousal was later shown to be a "reflex" due to stimulation of chemoreceptors and nociceptors, and not a direct effect of histamine on the central nervous system.

Speculatively, however, it is possible that the increased evoked potentials also involve primary extrapyramidal tracts, or that the exogenous histamine directly affects one of the extra-blood-brain-barrier brain structures, the functions of which are still obscure. Finally, it is well-documented that tension and stress exacerbate the symptoms of Tourette's syndrome, and control of an allergic reaction could contribute to the control of the symptoms in this patient.

Case 10 exhibits a symptom which is seldom mentioned in the bibliography. The phenomenon of compulsive obscene finger movements seems a logical extension of Tourette symptomatology in an environment where these finger signs are commonly used. Again, this "copropraxia" suggests a psychogenic component, as yet unspecified. It would appear that Itard's statement in 1825 about the etiology of coprolalia could apply here: When a tiqueur realizes that he has little if any control over his vocalizations and movements, concern over the nature of these involuntary actions "somehow" causes their worst expression to appear. Still, after almost 150 years, that "somehow" still eludes us.

FOLLOW-UP DATA ON PREVIOUSLY REPORTED CASES [4]

Case 1

This white male (G.E.), now 38 years old, was seen several times during 1971. In January he reported that he had lost his job of 15 months because of motor symptoms and coprolalia. He was suffering from head and leg tics along with "fuck you" exclamations in paroxysms 40 times a day. He had been taking chlordiazepoxide (Librium), 25 mg three times daily, refusing haloperidol because of drowsiness, dry mouth, gastrointestinal irritation, and loss of libido.

In February, the patient was willing to try haloperidol, and haloperidol was prescribed, 5 mg at bedtime, with amantadine HC1 (Symmetrel) 100 mg twice daily, while chlordiazepoxide was discontinued. When last seen in April, 1971, the patient showed at least 50 per cent improvement with this regimen, and the dose of amantadine HC1 was decreased to 100 mg in the morning.

Case 2

This white female patient (D.W.) has been seen about once every three months during 1970 and 1971. In March, 1970, the patient was still experiencing occasional tics, mainly when she was upset. A head tic and "yuck" vocalizations occurred about once a week. Her progress in school had been average except for an "F" in science, for which she went to summer school. School attendance has been poor, presumably due to her symptoms. She was 5 feet, 2 inches tall (157.5 cm) and weighed 115 lbs (52.3 kg), slightly overweight for her height.

In July, 1970, the patient was still overweight and an eyeblinking tic had become more frequent. Her dosage of haloperidol was increased to 2 mg three times daily. In December, her school progress had improved, although, after a transient improvement, her tics and vocalizations still troubled her about once a week.

In March, 1971, an occasional slight grunt in her voice was noted, along with tics in the face and arms. For three days she was tried on 4 mg of haloperidol three times daily with no improvement. Her height at this time was 5 feet, 5 inches (165.1 cm) and weight, 149 lbs (67.2 kg). She has been maintained on 2 mg haloperidol three times daily.

Case 3

Gradual reduction in haloperidol with good control of symptoms typified the course of treatment for this 10-year-old white male patient (J.S.) during 1970. He is currently in the fourth grade and doing well, except for math. He started "clearing his throat" in October, but this subsided without any increase in his medications.

This patient was last seen in December, 1970, when he was 10 years old, 50 inches tall (127 cm) and weighed 56½ lbs (25.7 kg). He is currently maintained on 4 mg haloperidol twice daily and benztropine mesylate (Cogentin), 0.25 mg per day.

Case 4

This white female patient (L.P.) is now 22 years old. Long-standing marital conflicts led to a separation from her husband in June, 1970, and a divorce the following December. As reported previously, she had a stillbirth in June of 1969 due to a strangulated cord and placenta previa. She has been maintained on haloperidol, 4 mg daily, with dextroamphetamine to combat drowsiness. Her vocal and muscular tics have been under moderate control, except when she is tired or anxious.

She had been attending a business school until her welfare payments were cut. Presently she is searching for a job, few of which are available in her town at the present time. She complains of no side effects, but has gained considerable weight in the last year.

Case 5

This white male patient (S.H.) is now in sixth grade and has been maintained on haloperidol, 5 mg per day. Good control of motor symptoms has been maintained, with occasional throat clearing or forced expiration. School problems necessitate special tutorials, and transfer to a special education school is being considered.

Case 6

This white male patient (G.A.) remains hospitalized in the same state hospital to which he was committed in 1960. No haloperidol has been prescribed, and symptoms of Tourette's syndrome are not prominent.

Case 7

This white female patient (L.E.), now 30 years old, was admitted to the psychiatric ward of a local hospital in March, 1971. Prior to this time, she had been taking no medications and had not been seen by us for about two years. She had seen a psychotherapist on occasion during that time, and apparently had managed to review the previous impressions of the senior author, one of which suggested that she didn't really want to lose her tic. As a result, she was very antagonistic to the interviewer and wished that "when the tic leaves me, it will go to (the senior author) or one of his kids."

Upon admission she was given a battery of psychotropic drugs with no improvement of vocal tics (a seal-like bark) or muscular tics of the upper extremities. Three days later haloperidol was prescribed (1 mg four times daily) and diphenhydramine (Benadryl), 50 mg four times daily. Later, some improvement was noted when the haloperidol dosage was raised to 2 mg four times daily, but complaints of drowsiness and a dry mouth led to a reduction of the dosage to the original level. Slight improvement was described on her discharge summary, and she is currently being maintained with haloperidol at the same dose.

Her IQ on the Shipley-Hartford scale was 95, and an EEG on March 15, 1971 was normal. The MMPI showed a paranoid element of sensitivity and hostility, and impulse controls appeared to be poor.

SUMMARY

Four new case histories of Gilles de la Tourette's syndrome are presented, along with follow-up reports on seven previously published case histories. One of these four new patients suffered from allergy, and subsequently a seasonal pattern of varying severity of Tourette symptoms was observed. Although the theories of Snyder[430] as to the etiology of the syndrome are attractive, the possibility of an histaminergic component is further substantiated by the well-documented pattern of symptom exacerbation concomitant with infectious disease. A rare symptom was present in another case, so-called "copropraxia," or involuntary obscene finger movements. Compulsive spitting is a more frequent form of copropraxia found in the syndrome.

Gilles de la Tourette's Syndrome. Volume 1: International Registry, p. 43-46, edited by F. Abuzzahab Sr. and F. Anderson. Mason Publishing Co., St. Paul ©1976.

A CASE OF GILLES DE LA TOURETTE'S SYNDROME IN HUNGARY

Laszlo Ivan, M.D.
The Second Clinic of Neurology and Psychiatry,
Medical University
Budapest, Hungary

The rarity of Gilles de la Tourette's syndrome is such that a review of published case reports is the only feasible method of surveying the broad aspects of the condition. The syndrome was originally described by Itard in 1825[232] and later differentiated and named as a syndrome by Gilles de la Tourette in 1885.[198] Among 2500 patients, Koster[255] in 1899 discovered two cases admitted to a neuropsychiatric hospital in Leipzig. Since that time, cases have been reported from Switzerland (1950), Poland (1958), France (1961), Canada (1962), Turkey, Finland, Great Britain and the United States.

Fernando[167] in 1967 summarized the 69 published case reports (18 female and 51 male) in a review and reported four new cases. However, he did not include the first case from Hungary reported at the Eighth International Congress of Neurology in Vienna in September, 1965.[233] (Since that time, the author has seen 3 additional cases in Hungary). A report of the first case follows, which is the first in the world literature to be treated with electroshock.

CASE REPORT

This male patient (I.P.) was admitted to our clinic in 1961 at age 20, exhibiting multiple generalized motor tics involving mainly the face, shoulders, arms and lower limbs, and also echopraxia, echolalia, coprolalia, and clicking and sucking noises. The motor tics had begun with grimace-like facial tics when the patient was 7, without any known antecedents. The patient was an only child. There was no family history of mental illness or tics, and home and school environments were satisfactory with good parental and social relations. Within a month after facial tics appeared, the motor tics had become multiple and generalized. He was hospitalized in a neuropsychiatric institute at this time and treated with barbiturates, chlorpromazine, phenothiazine, and other tranquilizers, as well as psychotherapy, all of which were ineffective. During this hospitalization he developed a varicella infection, after which verbal symptoms (echolalia, coprolalia) and echopraxia first appeared. Diagnosis was parainfectious encephalitis at this time. The symptoms continued unabated, and although the patient remained a lively, amenable, warmhearted boy, he became progressively more socially isolated because of his symptoms. His intelligence was above average and he graduated from secondary school with excellent marks.

When admitted to our clinic at age 20, he was a tall, thin man with no physical or laboratory findings except a thoracic scoliosis. Neurologic examination showed left central facial weakness, right hypoglossal weakness, polykinetic tendon reflexes of the lower limbs, slightly increased spastic muscle tone, and increased muscle excitability. The EEG was abnormal, with continuous and paroxysmal theta waves and spike-like bursts. A trial of anticonvulsive drugs did not affect the EEG. A lumbar pneumoencephalogram showed a somewhat more basal cisternal development of gracile and asymmetric ventricles.

The patient was depressed and dysphoric and socially isolated. Psychomotor activity was accelerated, and tics appeared intermittently, provoked by any kind of stress and fatigue. Sexual libido was slightly above average. Sleep was very light and marked by frightening dreams; the patient woke fatigued.

Because all other therapeutic attempts had failed, we tried electroshock therapy, giving 53 shock treatments over a period of 32 days (4 convulsions daily for 2 days, 3 convulsions daily for 13 days, and 2 convulsions daily for 3 days). The daily convulsions were repeated before the post-convulsion awakening. During the first few days of treatment, the patient remained fully oriented, and coprolalia returned during the post-convulsion period. Defrontalization (amnestic syndrome) did not occur until the fifteenth day of shock treatment and lasted until the 26th day. During this period, the patient showed violent psychomotor excitation for a few days, during which he would compulsively and agitatedly pack his suitcase, wait for the streetcar, etc. However, Tourette's symptoms ceased completely. By the 26th day, he had recovered from defrontalization, but coprolalia reappeared, so further electroshocks were given. By the 32nd day, the patient was clinically well. Follow-up 6 months later found him without any symptoms.

DISCUSSION

The causes of this very rare disease are not yet clear. There is little evidence to suggest that this syndrome is a disease entity with specific etiology. We know from the neuropsychiatric literature that Tourette's syndrome can follow Sydenham's chorea[89] and, in fact, practically all variations of symptoms short of the full syndrome can follow chorea.[112 273 355] Tourette's syndrome has also been seen after encephalitis lethargica[59] and in obsessional psychogenic disorders and compulsive shouting, as in Benedek's "Klazomania".[28] The typical preventive mechanisms and obsessional symptoms not infrequently can occur in schizophrenic illness.[11 300 436]

The view that the illness is an obsessive neurosis[11 19] is too limited. Heuscher[221] suggested that the tics are not a defense against an underlying psychosis. Suppressed hostility to parents or other significant persons has been suggested as the underlying psychodynamic by Ascher[11] and by Eisenberg,[152] Schneck,[410] Dunlap,[149] and Faux[161] noted the significance of the environmental feedback of rejection. The possibility of organic causation is suggested by the frequency of abnormal EEGs and of family histories of tics. Brain[59] described the tics as a sequel of encephalitis lethargica, which could affect the basal ganglia. It is noteworthy that the phenothiazine derivatives act in this area (Bockner's two cases[45] described in 1959, responded very promptly to chlorpromazine). Other patients seem to benefit from neuroleptic drugs, which probably act on the basal ganglia.[235 372] MacDonald[289] suggested that functional factors act on a substratum of organic brain damage, while Eisenberg[151] felt that the behavior of brain-damaged children can be affected by social factors. The only positive autopsy finding in a case of Gilles de la Tourette's syndrome showed an immature cell structure of the striatum on microscopic examination.[97]

Our opinion and suggestion is the same as MacDonald's[289] that Gilles de la Tourette's syndrome is the reaction of an unstable, immature (sometimes pathologically damaged) system to stimuli of an overwhelming nature. The usual regulative functions have not developed or have broken down and the system is prone to uncontrolled discharge.

SUMMARY

The first case of Gilles de la Tourette's syndrome reported from Hungary is described. This male patient first developed motor tics at age 7, and vocal tics (echolalia, coprolalia) after an attack of varicella somewhat later. Various drugs and psychotherapy were tried without effect, and symptoms continued unabated till age 20, when a course of 53 electroshock treatments over a period of 32 days resulted in complete cessation of symptoms. Various theories of the etiology of Tourette's syndrome are discussed. An explanation suggesting overwhelming stimuli impinging on an unstable, immature organism which lacks the usual regulative functions is favored.

Gilles de la Tourette's Syndrome. Volume 1: International Registry, p. 47-67, edited by F. Abuzzahab Sr. and F. Anderson. Mason Publishing Co., St. Paul ©1976.

EXPERIENCE IN 20 CASES OF TOURETTE'S SYNDROME

Richard L. Jenkins, M.D.,
and
Barry N. Fine, M.D.
Department of Psychiatry,
University of Iowa
Iowa City, Iowa 52240 U.S.A.

Our series included 12 boys and 6 girls. Median age of onset was 7 years with a range of from 4 to 15. The evaluation was at an age range from 7 to 25 with a median age of 12. The age range at follow-up of 18 cases was from 10 to 37 with a median age of 19. Follow-up periods ranged from 6 months to 16 years with a median of 7 years. Thirteen patients had clear coprolalia, and 7 were without coprolalia.

At the follow-up, 4 patients were symptom free; 3 of these were on no medication, and 1 was on 2 mg of haloperidol daily. Seven patients had good control of tics or very minor symptoms. Six were on haloperidol, 2½ to 6 mg daily, and 1 was on no medication. Four patients had some tics. Two were on no medication, 1 was on 6 mg haloperidol daily, and the last on 20 mg of trifluoperazine and 250 mg of diphenhydramine daily.

We have used haloperidol in 15 of our 20 cases. In 13 of these cases (cases 2, 3, 4, 5, 6, 12, 13, 15, 16, 17, 18, 19, and 20) it was of benefit, usually giving complete or almost complete control of symptoms. The patient in case 16 discontinued medication because of side effects despite good control of the tics. We have had no case of Tourette's disease in which haloperidol did not reduce or control the tics. In an additional case (Case 14) the tics had disappeared before haloperidol was given, and this medication was without benefit to the torticollis (see case description below). Methedrine had an unfavorable effect on the tics in Case 6. Both dextroamphetamine and methylphenidate made the symptoms worse in Case 19. Dextroamphetamine administered in Case 20 was followed by exacerbation of the tics. Dextroamphetamine was administered also in Case 16 but was discontinued for lack of benefit. Thus, we have some evidence that cerebral stimulants increase the tics.

The first four cases in this series have been reported previously with the same case numbers.[84 88] Two more were reported by Dr. James Chapel.[86] (His Case 1 is our Case 4, and his Case 2 is our Case 12). Twelve of our 20 cases of Tourette's syndrome have been previously reported. Here we present follow-up data on 10 of these 12 cases (Cases 8 and 11 were not available for follow-up) and data on 8 new cases. Case 21, which we do not regard as a case of Tourette's syndrome, is included for comparison.

In all our cases, substantial family pathology was evident. It usually appeared that one parent was an overly rigid, demanding, punitive, and/or rejecting person, while the other parent seemed to be endeavoring to make up to the child for this severity and over-critical attitude. The child became in some sense the focus of the parental conflict and in some instances, at least, began to use his symptoms consciously as a weapon against the severe parent. Clearly it is important to seek to reduce or ameliorate the family conflict in cases of Tourette's disease, or failing this, to remove the child from the conflicted situation in order to make possible some effective control of the symptoms.

Case 1

At the age of 7, this boy (W.Z., B.D. 4-6-47) began having facial tics with blinking of the eyes and jerking of the arms, shoulders, and neck, which progressed in the next two years to tics of the entire body. Inarticulate cries also began to develop, becoming coprolalic words by the age of twelve. In the next four years, numerous treatment efforts included hypnosis, deconditioning with shock, and at least 40 different drugs, but the only improvement seemed to be on an interpersonal basis.

In 1962 (age 15) neurological examination and EEG were within normal limits and IQ was around 90. The patient was begun on haloperidol with almost complete remission of his symptoms at a dose of 6.3 mg per day. When medication was discontinued in 1963 because of abnormal laboratory tests symptoms returned. Haloperidol (4.5 mg daily) was reinstituted about a month later without problems, and the patient was followed on an outpatient basis for the next 3 years on doses of between 3 and 4 mg per day. This dosage was somewhat less than the optimum, but the patient's symptoms were reasonably well controlled with no side effects. Symptoms were more pronounced during periods of anger or conflict with his family and improved during periods of relative calm.

The patient was seen in March, 1970 (age 22), for follow-up after essentially no contact for four years. He exhibited motor tics, particularly tapping of his thigh, grunting noises, and mild coprolalia. He described a sporadic work record in the years since he had left school including six jobs during the past year, and he reported also a continuation of conflict in his parental home, where he still lived. The patient reported he had been taking 4 mg of haloperidol daily for the past two years plus chlorpromazine, 25 mg b.i.d. He reported some symptoms of sleepiness and also a weight gain of 25 pounds in the previous year.

The patient was asked to discontinue chlorpromazine, to increase his haloperidol to 6 mg daily, and to add benztropine mesylate (Cogentin), ½ mg b.i.d. After approximately two weeks, the patient reported that he was no longer sleepy but complained that benztropine mesylate made his mouth extremely dry. This side effect disappeared when benztropine was discontinued. The patient felt that his tics were decreased somewhat on the higher dose (6 mg) of haloperidol but did admit to being under tremendous pressure with "$5 in my pocket and $5 in the bank and no job."

Ater 2½ weeks, it appeared to the psychiatrist that motor tics were less frequent and that the grunting noises were fewer and dropped away during the interview. The patient was asked to raise his dose to 8 mg haloperidol daily.

At contact about one month later, the patient reported that he had reduced his dosage to 4 mg daily after only 2 days at 8 mg because he became quite sleepy, but that on this lower dosage he felt that the improvement he had noticed on 3 mg b.i.d. had been gradually lost. The patient agreed to again try 3 mg b.i.d. and is presently on this dosage.

Case 2

At age seven, this boy (P.B., B.D. 7-10-53) developed mild facial tics, some occasional protrusions of the tongue, and jerking movements of the arms, along with the vocal expletives "Ha", "Arf," and "Meow." All symptoms were more pronounced when he was under stress. At school he was rowdy, stubborn, and prone to temper tantrums, and this behavior as much as his distracting tics, caused his exclusion from school in 1962 at age nine. At that time he was evaluated in our clinic and exhibited the tics described above with the addition of the words "shit" and "fuck," barking, grinding of teeth, and compulsive touching. EEG and physical examinations were within normal limits. His full scale WISC IQ was 107. He showed no improvement after 13 sessions of psychotherapy and a trial of primidone (Mysoline). Haloperidol was begun in early 1963, and improvement was noted in 48 hours with a reduction to four tics daily when he was discharged 11 days later on 1½ mg haloperidol per day. Few side effects could be observed.

The patient was followed on an outpatient basis from 1963 until September, 1965. Four weeks after discharge, his tics were completely controlled on 2 mg haloperidol daily. There was some restlessness and muscle stiffness, but benztropine mesylate was not given. A number of attempts were made to reduce the dosage of medication to 1 mg daily, but on each occasion symptoms returned. On one occasion when the medication was reduced to 1 mg haloperidol daily, the parents reported blinking and flapping of the hands which ceased when the medication was again raised to 2 mg twice daily.

After no contact for almost four years, the family physician reported that the patient, who was at that time on 3 mg haloperidol daily, had become rather sleepy in class. The medication was reduced to 2 mg per day, and the patient became less sleepy with no return of tics. In December, 1969 (age 16), he began to feel nervous and experienced some blinking of the eyes. Increase of haloperidol to 2½ mg daily controlled nervousness and blinking.

In March, 1970, the patient was seen for re-evaluation. He was then a junior in high school and receiving C and D grades. His symptoms were fairly well controlled at that time, but benztropine mesylate, ½ mg b.i.d., was tried for control of possible side effects (slight muscle stiffness). This was discontinued because of increased dryness of the mouth. Because the patient reported that he was somewhat more nervous than usual, haloperidol dosage was raised from 2 mg per day to 2½ mg per day. The patient reported that this seemed to make him feel less nervous although perhaps slightly more sleepy. At the present time there are still no symptoms of Tourette's syndrome.

Case 3

At age 10 this boy (D.S., B.D. 8-31-49) developed a hiccuping tic which was high-pitched and whooping. Over the next three years sudden squatting and extension and retraction of the arms appeared. In the next year he developed a grabbing motion directed at his mother's breasts, accompanied by the vocal expletives "tits" and "titties." The last tics to appear were coprolalic utterances of "shit," "God dammit," and "flutchy nay."(The patient explained that this was French for fornication). The patient had been in psychotherapy for four years, but the condition had become progressively worse, and he was admitted to our hospital for evaluation and treatment in 1963 at age 13. On our ward he was observed to have approximately 106 tics per day with a verbal to motor ratio of 10 to 1. Neurological examination was normal and the WISC placed him in the normal range of intelligence.

The patient was placed on haloperidol. His motor tics disappeared when dosage reached 6 mg daily and vocal tics vanished in the next few days. On discharge from the hospital in September, 1963, the parents felt that his medication had not been "stabilized" because he was quite sleepy and drooled. In retrospect, it appears he might have benefited from a drug such as benztropine mesylate, but this was not given. Two years later, his parents were well pleased with the control of his symptoms and stated that only under stress were there two or three disguised and very mild tics per day.

At follow-up in 1970 when the patient was 20, the parents stated that the dosage had been somewhat lower in the fall of 1966 when the patient entered his senior year of high school, with symptoms well controlled, and during 1966-67 the dosage was gradually lowered without return of symptomatology. At graduation from high school the patient was off all medication, and symptoms were only very occasionally noted. The patient entered a junior college but dropped out and "laid around the house for six months." He then took a job in a supermarket but was unhappy and unexpectedly enlisted in the army engineering corps where, according to the parents, he was just barely accepted. After five months he was sent to Vietnam where he served a full one-year tour of duty. The patient became a corporal in the army and was to be discharged in the summer of 1970. So far as the parents are aware, there is no problem with Tourette's syndrome. The patient was home from his tour in Vietnam for 1 month in winter, 1970, and the parents report no major symptoms, no coprolalia, and only two or three little hiccups noted during that month. At present the patient continues in the army and is on no medication with almost complete remission of his symptoms.

Case 4

This girl, (D.J.H., B.D. 11-12-51) developed tics consisting of the vocal expletive "yeah, yeah pooh" after a traumatic tonsillectomy in 1956 at age five. Soon chest pounding, then barking, then jerking of the neck, and other tics followed. She could stop them when she wanted to, but another "habit" replaced each tic as quickly as she discarded it. During the next six years the tics waxed and waned in frequency and became a real problem only at age 12 (in 1964) when she was excluded from school. Chlordiazepoxide (Librium) was tried at this time without improvement.

When admitted to our hospital about six months later, at age 12, she exhibited high-pitched clearing of the throat accompanied by facial grimaces, screwing up of the eyes, and unilateral shrugging of her shoulder with flailing of the arm on that side at a rate of about 200 per hour during waking hours but greatly decreased during sleep. The parents also described coprolalia consisting mostly of the words "fuck," "shit," and "son of a bitch." These vocal tics were often non-obscene but closely resembled an obscene word, and the patient candidly admitted to having mental coprolalia whenever she said "shoot" or "son of a bitch." The patient would also grasp and pinch nearby persons, which she said was part of the tic, but observers felt this to be in great part a deliberately hostile gesture. The neurological examination and EEG were normal and the full-scale WISC IQ was 80. She was found to be a very selfish, domineering, and spoiled child. She feared growing up, was afraid of menstruation, of rape, and of sex in general. She improved dramatically for 48 hours while on a placebo but soon relapsed. On haloperidol the improvement was equally as rapid but was sustained. She was discharged in August, 1964, on haloperidol, 5.2 mg daily, with symptoms well-controlled.

Shortly after discharge, there was some evidence of stiffness and gross tremors in both hands, but benztropine mesylate was not prescribed. The haloperidol was reduced to 4.8 mg daily, and about this time the patient began to gain substantial weight. A further reduction in dosage to 3.2 mg daily was not sufficient to control facial grimacing and some clicking of the teeth. At interview in 1965, when the patient was on the 3.2 mg, there was no evidence of tics, but the patient said she had some verbal and motor tics at home.

From 1965 through 1967 the medication was gradually reduced to about 1 mg per day with increasing return of symptoms. In 1967 (age 16) the medication was gradually raised, and symptoms were brought under better control.

At re-evaluation in March, 1970, the patient stated that for the past two years she has been taking 2 mg haloperidol twice daily. There was still some evidence of tics, particularly facial grimacing and some sniffing in the morning with coprolalia very infrequent. The patient finds this to be somewhat embarrassing although she says it does not impede her work in school, where she hopes to graduate from a work-study program which includes training as a child-care worker for mentally retarded children. She will receive a high school diploma at the end of the year.

The patient herself was neatly groomed, well-dressed, well-composed, and extremely pleasant, a dramatic change from the behavior at age 12. The parents confirmed that she was doing well in her schooling and they were pleased with her general life adjustment.

Haloperidol dosage was raised from 4 mg to 5 mg daily with no additional side effects, and then to 6 mg daily. At this dosage level, symptoms decreased significantly, sleepiness was not increased, and there were no other signs of side effects.

Case 5

This male patient (P.S.J., B.D. 2-23-40) began having facial tics at age 10 or 11, soon followed by tongue protrusion, frequent shrugging of the shoulders, stomping of the foot, jerking of the right or left arm, and slapping of the right leg. All of these motor tics were accompanied by mental swearing and all disappeared after one year, tending to reoccur only when he was under stress. At age 22, his tics reappeared with the addition of barking, coughing, and the vocal expletive "shit." Past history indicates his birth was illegitimate and that his mother was institutionalized for mental illness when he was four years of age. He was raised by his grandparents, who were strict, rigid people with high expectations.

He was seen in our hospital in 1963 and was admitted in 1964. Neurological examination revealed no pathology. EEG was normal. He had a full-scale WAIS IQ of 99. His performance on projective tests implied an inability to experience warm feelings toward people and a hostility toward females with a fear of retaliation.

His tics on the ward were charted at the rate of two or three a minute and coughing or barking with the same frequency. With haloperidol, there was a rapid decrease to four or five disguised coprolalic utterances and a few minor facial tics per day. He was discharged after three weeks and was followed on an outpatient basis. When seen in March of 1965, he was on 4 mg of haloperidol daily and was having one or two coprolalic utterances per week. He had returned to his previous job of grave-digging, which he had lost because of his disability.

In March, 1970, the patient reported by telephone that he was out of work and no longer taking medication because it made him too sleepy even on lower doses. He stated that the coughing tics and some of the motor tics had come back since he stopped medication. He was aware that the medication helped him but was concerned about the side effects. The patient refused a return visit to the clinic.

Case 6

This girl (H.S., B.D. 4-2-49) first developed tics at age six when she began to blink her eyes and twitch her face. The tics were mild and not a source of worry to the parents. At age nine after an attack of measles the tics increased in intensity. Very soon tongue protrusion and some shoulder jerks also appeared. A barking cough developed at age 10, but disappeared following a tonsillectomy. The syndrome progressively worsened until December of 1961 (age 12) when the patient refused to leave home for school and frequently refused even to get out of bed. Private psychiatrists were consulted. She has had a total of approximately 25 psychotherapy sessions without improvement.

When she was admitted to our hospital in early 1962, the parents, and especially the father, were found to be difficult to work with. He was rather a perfectionistic, demanding, critical, and rigid individual, while the mother was passive, nervous, and kowtowed to her husband. The patient failed to show improvement, and after three months she was removed by her father against medical advice and admitted to a private hospital in another state. Her father removed her from that hospital after four months because of her lack of improvement. Readmission to that hospital for a second four months did produce a good result, however, since she established a good relationship with her psychiatrist and became able to control her tics while sitting in his office. Gradually she was able to extend this control and left the hospital much improved. In the meantime, our department, not knowing of this improvement in the child, contacted the parents and offered them a trial of haloperidol, which they accepted because she was still showing some tics, particularly in church. When seen on this occasion in our hospital, the patient was found to have few tics. Neurological examination and EEG were within normal limits, and the full-scale WISC IQ was 112.

The patient was started on haloperidol without any change obvious to the hospital staff, but the father was sure that her tics were better controlled. She was discharged in 1963 after about six weeks in the hospital and followed for regular outpatient visits, returning to school in spite of extreme shyness and inhibition. The patient reported that when haloperidol was withheld from her for about 48 hours on one occasion, the tics returned with greater intensity and frequency but were quickly brought under control when haloperidol was reinstituted.

After an absence of 3 years from our clinic, the patient and her parents were seen again in March, 1970 (age 20), and expressed grave doubts as to whether the haloperidol did, in fact, produce any beneficial results. The patient felt that she had improved before her second admission to our hospital and that the haloperidol did not relieve her Tourette's symptoms to any extent. The patient's uncertainty about the benefits of haloperidol is certainly understandable because she was given little understanding of Tourette's syndrome by those she saw and psychiatrists and physicians made contradictory statements regarding "organic factors," "emotional aspects," "a condition like encephalitis," and "a condition like epilepsy."

The patient in 1970 was an extremely attractive, well-groomed, and intelligent young woman. The only noticeable tics were blinking of the eyes. The patient stated that she had done well in high school, finishing the previous year with A and B grades. She worked for a time as a psychiatric aide but in November, because of many conflicts at home, because she was particularly tired due to the high dose of haloperidol (16 mg per day), and certain other reasons, she sought help from a psychiatrist who hospitalized her at that time. The patient was given much supportive psychotherapy, total milieu therapy, and amobarbital (Amytal) interviews and taken off haloperidol completely. There was no increase in her blink-like tics and she was no longer as tired as she had been in the past. The patient did note, interestingly enough, that when the psychiatrist added small doses of methamphetamine to the amobarbital, her symptoms returned in much greater intensity for a day or two. This occurred a number of times in spite of her requests that the addition of methamphetamine be discontinued. When the psychiatrist finally agreed, there was no recurrence of the symptoms of Tourette's syndrome during amobarbital interviews.

With cessation of extreme sleepiness, after discontinuing haloperidol, the patient entered the local area community college and is presently taking 9 hours of credits. She hopes to enter a regular college next year, possibly a small college where she expects to be more comfortable and is thinking in terms initially of a bachelor's degree but perhaps a master's degree after that. Her expectations are quite appropriate for her intellectual and academic abilities.

On March 20, 1970, the patient agreed to undergo another trial of haloperidol. She first discontinued the dose of perphenazine, 8 mg daily, which had been prescribed by her psychiatrist. By April 4 she was taking 4 mg of haloperidol daily with no evidence of side effects or sleepiness, but was once again eating excessively, a side effect which had plagued her previously when taking haloperidol. She stated that the one remaining symptom of eye-blinking showed no improvement. The patient agreed to increase her medication to 8 mg haloperidol daily from 4 mg daily. When she reported two weeks later, she indicated that after three days on the higher dose, she had noticed that she was becoming quite sleepy and therefore discontinued the haloperidol completely. When she stopped the haloperidol, the sleepiness stopped, and even after two weeks of taking no haloperidol, she noticed no increase in her very slight tic symptom. The patient was told that there appeared to be little point in taking haloperidol and that she could continue with the perphenazine, 8 mg daily, as required, according to the instructions of her local psychiatrist. In view of the lack of response to 8 mg of haloperidol, the patient was once again quite convinced that haloperidol had never really helped her very much, although she agreed in retrospect that perhaps it had been of some value during times of stress when the symptoms might otherwise have been exacerbated. It is interesting that the patient reports that her symptoms of Tourette's syndrome increase during times of relaxation, such as when watching television, but cease almost completely when she is actively engaged in some activity, particularly studying or working on academic papers. The patient's final question to the psychiatrist at our clinic was how she might relax more, because this did seem to help her symptoms sometimes. She was told, not entirely with tongue in cheek, that probably the best way to relax would be to avoid psychiatrists for a time, to make preparations to attend college on a full-time basis, away from the conflict in her home situation, and to attempt to avoid all medication including both haloperidol and perphenazine if at all possible, and certainly not to involve herself with hypnosis or psychotherapy as had been suggested recently. In essence, she was encouraged to relax by concentrating on developing her own life style rather than concentrating on psychiatric treatment.

Case 7

While in kindergarten, this girl (L.Y., B.D. 2-28-57) developed head-jerking which was replaced, in rapid succession, by blinking, then stamping of her foot, then jumping on one foot. More recently the tic was described as a jerking from the neck and shoulders with an occasional verbal tic. Her physician prescribed hydroxyzine (Vistaril) three times daily without success. Chiropractic treatments from two different chiropractors were fruitless. In late 1964 (age 7) the child was seen in our clinic and exhibited the following tics: A pecking motion of the head and neck and a sudden spasm of one side or all of the body resembling a reaction to an electric shock. An accompanying inarticulate vocal tic was infrequent. Neurological examination at that time was normal. The EEG was within normal limits. Full-scale WISC IQ was 113. The diagnosis of Tourette's syndrome was made, but the parents refused to accept treatment. The mother was described as a strict, demanding person who expected peak performance from this adopted child. The father was passive and willing to go along with the mother in order to keep the peace. The child seemed to be a nervous, angry, and inhibited young girl who was reacting strongly to her mother.

The parents were contacted again in March, 1970, when the patient was 13 years of age and average student in grade 7. The mother stated that there had been no motor or vocal tics of any kind since early 1965. After refusal of medical treatment in 1964, the patient was seen by a chiropractor for about two months twice weekly and then once weekly for a time after that. Within two months, the tics seemed to drop away.

The patient's local doctor agreed with our suggestion that chiropractic treatment might well have taken the pressure off the child by placing her problem on an organic basis and de-emphasizing the emotional aspects.

Note: Cases 8 and 11 were not available for follow-up.

Case 9

At age four, this male patient (R.P., B.D. 12-13-33) developed a slight jerking of the hands and trunk associated with a high, barking sound. These movements later spread to other parts of the body and at times were so violent that he was "thrown" or fell with these spells. They were present during light sleep but disappeared in sound sleep. He was seen at the Iowa University Hospital in 1948 (age 15) and diagnosed as having myoclonic epilepsy. A sodium amytal interview with strong direct suggestions to "cease his tics" was unfruitful.

He was admitted to our hospital in 1958 at age 25. He stated that his illness had waxed and waned for the past 20 years but was now simply "wearing him down." He had coprolalia, barking, and various motor tics. He admitted no peace from his afflictions except during sound sleep or during sexual intercourse. Neurological examination and EEG were normal. Psychological test studies suggested a poor masculine identification. After four months of unsuccessful intensive therapy, he asked to be discharged from the hospital against medical advice. He has not been seen since, but his family described him as having a rather erratic life pattern and tending to become involved in antisocial behavior. At the father's last contact with the patient five years ago (1965, age 32), he continued to have symptoms described above, but he reported to his sister in 1969 that he no longer had as severe a problem with his motor and vocal tics. He also indicated that he had written some bad checks, and he is presently an inmate of the Colorado State Penitentiary.

Case 10

While in a foster home at age nine, this boy (R.O.G., B.D. 2-14-45) began having facial twitches which were followed in three months by verbal tics. His condition was called St. Vitus' dance. He was returned home and soon lost his tics, only to have them reappear when he was returned to the foster home. When first seen in our hospital in 1957 at age 12, he had motor tics consisting of repetitive stretching of the neck to one side with associated grimacing, protrusion of the tongue, cracking of the knuckles, and assorted body jerks. There were frequent snortings, high-pitched clearing of the throat, and expletives of "nigger's ass," "fuck you," and "bitch, bitch, bitch," when his mother's name was mentioned. This symptomatology remitted, but never for very long, and he was admitted to our hospital in 1958 at age 13 for a period of six months. On reserpine and psychotherapy his tics decreased greatly and he was discharged to remain on reserpine for approximately one year. When interviewed in 1964 (age 19) he appeared free of tics except for occasional slight facial twitching or very rare muffled, inarticulate sounds. In view of the very slight evidence of symptoms, a trial of haloperidol was not felt to be warranted. The patient attributed the remission to his determination to control himself, and to the help and understanding given him by his high school wrestling coach. In February, 1970, the examining physician noted no evidence of any symptoms or signs of Tourette's syndrome. The patient seemed to be generally in good spirits with no evidence of emotional disturbance and reported no symptoms since his spontaneous recovery in 1964.

The patient graduated from high school in 1964 and entered college that same year to major in physical education. He attended college for about two and a half years and was on the wrestling team until he broke his leg. He continued to attend college with his leg in a hip cast for many months and left college after two and a half years, mostly for financial reasons. The patient has had a number of jobs since that time and has done reasonably well. Recently he had his draft classification changed from 4-F to 1-Y to make it easier to get certain kinds of jobs. He intends to marry shortly and has applied for a position with the highway patrol, but he still hopes to finish his college degree and to teach physical education in high school.

Case 12

When this 14-year-old boy (W.T., B.D. 1-11-51) had a tonsillectomy at age twelve, he was told postoperatively to sniff to keep his nostrils clear. He continued to sniff after he had completely healed, and within a month after the operation, developed the following tics: A twitching of his left shoulder, then his right shoulder, then a compulsion to stamp his left foot down hard on the floor; next, extension of his neck backwards and to the sides, all accompanied by an impulse to say obscene words. (This has been called "mental coprolalia"). Soon thereafter the mother noted that he often had a twitch accompanied by a "sort of a hop and step" when he walked. Nine months later vocal expletives and a barking cough developed. Very soon the vocal tics became coprolalic ("fuck" and "shit," with "Jesus" and "Christ" less frequent).

Osteopathic and chiropractic treatment failed. He was placed on medication which included, successively, hydroxyzine, diphenylhydantoin, phenobarbital, and chlordiazepoxide without any improvement. When seen in our hospital in mid-1965 at age 14, this patient exhibited all of the tics mentioned above. Neurological examination including EEG were within normal limits. He had a full-scale WISC IQ of 78.

The mother, an aggressive person, had been separated from her husband since 1962 (when the patient was 11) because of "inability to agree on the management of the children." In spite of the separation, the father spent all of his days-off on the farm with the family, brought home his paycheck, bought groceries, and, in fact, lived at home except that every night at 9:00 p.m. he left to sleep at the home of a nearby relative. This situation was complicated by the presence of a 43-year-old salesman who brought his accounts to the farm to be checked by the mother. This man behaved much more like a father toward the family than did the natural father. He was well liked by all. However, the patient resented him and also resented the fact that his mother worked long hours in a restaurant and a department store. He wanted her at home and his father back in his natural place, but the mother said that if the father came home to live, she would leave. In general, the boy was passive, disliked violence, and was unsure of himself. He also admitted to some guilt regarding masturbation and, all in all, was a very unhappy young man.

He was started on haloperidol and within two weeks, tics were rare. When last seen in July, 1965, he was well controlled on 2 mg daily and reported an average of one tic approximately every two weeks.

In December, 1968, on a dosage of 1½ mg haloperidol daily, some of the tics were recurring, particularly occasional noises in the throat and jerking of the shoulders. The medication was raised to 2½ mg daily and the symptoms cleared. In 1969 (age 18) the patient found that when he reduced the medication, the symptoms did not return unless he was particularly tired or under stress. At outpatient evaluation in March, 1970, the patient was in good spirits, appeared well-groomed, relaxed, and quite verbal. He said he had gained considerable weight in the three years on haloperidol and that about four months ago he had stopped taking medication completely. After about a week the tics began to return, increasing in severity over the next two weeks. After three weeks had passed with no medication, he resumed 2½ mg daily, and shortly thereafter the tics were again completely controlled except for occasional return of symptoms when he was tired. The patient reported some sleepiness when medication was first resumed, and also some muscle stiffness, particularly in the back of the neck.

The patient agreed to increase his haloperidol from 2½ mg daily to 3 mg daily in divided doses and to add benztropine mesylate ½ mg twice daily. After 4 weeks the patient reported that on the slightly higher dose of haloperidol he was more relaxed and that perhaps the tics were less likely to occur under pressure and when he was tired. He did feel more sleepy at work but was also sleeping better at night, and also indicated that within 2 or 3 days after he began taking the benztropine mesylate, muscle stiffness lessened.

Case 13

This adopted female child (B.M., B.D. 1-13-50) first began to develop tics accompanied by temper tantrums at about age 9, when she was in third grade. Tics progressed from head jerks to arms and then the entire body. At about age 11 or 12, she began to make grunting noises and barking sounds, and developed a hiccup-like vocal tic with jerking of her entire chest so severe that an entire church pew would jerk with the severity of the patient's motions. At about age 12, she went through a period of severe eye blinking and began to repeat such phrases as "I want, I want, I want." The parents described the child as a sensitive, tender-hearted girl who was especially attracted to children and older people, who was always very thoughtful and considerate, but who had been increasingly ostracized and teased by other children because of her affliction. The parents were rigid and inflexible individuals. The mother, a dominant, aggressive, and compulsive person, set very high standards for herself and her family, and the father was a rather ineffective but somewhat punitive parent who tended to be uninvolved in family problems.

This girl was admitted to the hospital for a stay of about 5 weeks at age 16 in June, 1966. The multiple motor and verbal tics described above were present, including stiffening of the legs, blinking of the eyes, frequent protrusions of the tongue, and a high-pitched sniffling and clearing of her throat. She was started on haloperidol. At a dose of 6 mg daily with 1 mg benztropine mesylate (Cogentin) twice daily there was good control of both motor and verbal tics. Remaining tics were much easier for her to control, and the patient felt more acceptable to her parents and to her peer groups.

At follow-up in March, 1970, the parents reported that the patient was doing well. She had graduated from high school the previous year and was working in her home town and living with friends in a girls' dormitory. The patient adjusts her medication between 3 mg and a maximum of 6 mg daily depending on the amount needed to control her symptoms. On the higher dose, she becomes somewhat sleepy, and after a period of good control, she lowers the dose to about 3 mg per day. If the symptoms return (usually slight blinking and some vocal grunting occasioned by periods of stress or pressure), the patient gradually increases medication until the symptoms are in control.

Case 14

This male patient (G.B., B.D. 8-3-43) was first admitted to our hospital in 1959 at age 15, because of a combination of vocal and motor tics which, in retrospect, are highly suggestive of Tourette's syndrome. Tics consisted of a peculiar cough, clearing of the throat, tic-like movements of the head, and gross undulating movements of the trunk and extremities. The patient was discharged after 6 months with a diagnosis of anxiety reaction and possible post-encephalitic syndrome secondary to mumps. The patient's own recollection of the course of illness after discharge is rather vague; apparently, after a time, the tics dropped away sufficiently to enable him to complete high school and obtain his bachelor's degree.

There were no further symptoms until 1969 (age 25) when the patient started to have tic-like movements of the head while undergoing the pressures of seeking a new job. He was hospitalized locally, received thioridazine (Mellaril) and later diazepam (Valium) with some benefit, but without further improvement and was referred to our hospital four months later. At that time there was constant repetitive jerking and turning of the head to the left with some stuttering when talking about emotion-laden topics. The impression was hysterical neurosis, conversion type. There was some evidence of spastic torticollis, but apparently the constant deviation to the left was not present when he was discharged about a month later. He was placed on diazepam, 10 mg three times daily while in the hospital, and this seemed to be of some benefit. One month after discharge, he was hospitalized again briefly in his home town because of increased tics and continuous spasms of the neck. He was placed on thioridazine, doxepin (Sinequan), and chlorphenesin carbamate (Maolate) with no apparent benefits.

At personal interview in March, 1970, the patient had been off all medication for two days with no worsening of his condition. There was definite deviation of the head to the left which he could not rectify. The patient was placed on haloperidol, which was gradually increased by ½ mg daily to a dosage of 3 mg per day plus ½ mg benztropine mesylate twice daily. At this dosage he reported that his neck seemed less stiff and the torticollis was perhaps loosening up, but the tics were returning again. Since there was little subsequent change at this dosage and he reported being a bit more nervous because he was looking for a job, he was asked to double the haloperidol dosage to 3 mg twice daily. However, there was no additional benefit after two weeks at this dosage and the patient felt his neck was now more stiff than before. The patient was advised to reduce the haloperidol to 2 mg daily and that if he noticed no worsening of his condition or perhaps some improvement, he might reduce the medication further, to 1-2 mg daily. Further follow-up is not yet available.

Case 15

This male patient (C.S., B.D. 8-11-58) was seen in our clinic in June, 1967, at age 8 for valuation of multiple tics. The patient first began to show tics at age 6. These began as blinking of the eyes and fine tremors of the hands, progressed to shaking of the head and shoulders, and finally involved the arms and entire body. There was also excessive clearing of the throat, which developed into guttural noises.

The patient appeared as a pleasant boy who smiled frequently, was easily excited, and appeared quite volatile and uninhibited, abruptly blurting out whatever came into his mind. During the interview, no tics or other symptoms of Tourette's syndrome were observed, but when the patient was left alone and observed via a one-way mirror, he displayed marked, almost convulsive, grimacing of the facial muscles, jerks of the right arm and then entire body, and he shouted unintelligibly. When the examiner returned, the patient was again able to control these symptoms. Neurological examination was within normal limits, and intellectual testing revealed borderline intelligence on repeated testing.

The patient was placed on haloperidol and showed marked improvement when he reached a dosage of 1.2 mg twice daily. After 3 months at this dosage, the family reported only minimal motor and verbal tics and much better relations with other children. A year later, the parents reported that the tics were returning. Medication was raised to 2 mg haloperidol twice daily, and tics were again brought under control.

In 1970 (at age 12) the patient's mother indicated that there were no motor or verbal tics on the continued dosage of 2 mg haloperidol plus ½ mg benztropine mesylate twice daily and that they were satisfied with the patient's condition. The patient was continuing in a special education class and expected to enter junior high school special education the next year.

Case 16

This male patient (N.A., B.D. 9-20-47) had shown various neurotic manifestations since early childhood involving nailbiting, nightmares, enuresis, feeding problems, and frequent fantasies involving sexuality and violence. Home and school adjustment had been poor, and the patient began to manifest various tics at about age 9, consisting of facial grimaces, head jerking, eye blinking, loud coughing, barking, abrupt inhaling, biting, and at times shouting of obscenities in a stuttering fashion. The patient had received psychotherapy, various tranquilizers, and phenobarbital without success. There was a history of conflict in the home environment. The father was domineering, argumentative and hostile, and the mother, rather dramatic, overprotective and inconsistent. The father had a habitual facial twitch and the mother a consistent habit of coughing and clearing her throat.

In 1967 at age 20 the patient was given a trial of haloperidol and received a maximum of 9 mg/day along with benztropine mesylate to control side effects. Apparently the tics were much reduced during this trial of haloperidol, but the patient discontinued haloperidol because of the side effects, which he called "inner driveness."

The patient was hospitalized in March, 1968, at which time he demonstrated the tics described above. Neurological examination and EEG were within the normal limits, and full scale IQ was 96. He was treated with amphetamine, diphenhydramine, and chlorpromazine with little improvement except on high doses of diphenhydramine and chlorpromazine. Two attempts at a retrial of haloperidol were unsuccessful because the patient refused to take it for more than 2 days for fear of the side effects he had experienced in 1967. The patient was discharged in July, 1968, on fairly high doses of diphenhydramine and chlorpromazine with partial improvement in his symptoms.

At follow-up in 1970 (age 23), the patient reported that Tourette's symptoms were still present to a moderate extent. For about one year after discharge, he had taken chlorpromazine, 500 mg daily, and diphenhydramine, 400 mg daily, the latter mainly to counteract the side effects of chlorpromazine. He was then switched to trifluoperazine (Stelazine) which he took off and on for the following year. In January, 1970, the patient began to take trifluoperazine, 20 mg a day, and diphenydramine, 250 mg a day.

Case 17

This girl (E.B., B.D. 11-25-58) was first seen for outpatient evaluation at age 7 in November, 1966. She appeared neatly dressed, smiled frequently, and generally was bashful and shy. Tics included jerking of the head from left to right, frequent blinking of the eyes and occasional jerking of the neck. When observed secretly while alone, she also made grunting sounds. Her parents stated that the patient had begun to shake her head and clear her throat excessively during the previous fall. Throat-clearing had developed into a deep guttural sound resembling a grunt which accompanied the tics and became increasingly louder as the months progressed. Head twitching and blinking of the eyes began gradually, accompanied by noticeable tics of the nose and mouth. The tics became more violent and progressively involved her shoulders and arms until at the time of evaluation her entire body was involved in jerks and tics. She also jumped up and down on both feet or stamped one foot, usually the right one. The tics occurred on the average of 4 to 5 times a minute, although they were absent while the patient slept. Under stress or excitement the symptoms were more violent.

Prior to onset of symptoms, the patient enjoyed being with people, was compliant and pleasant, and "almost a model child." At the time of evaluation, the parents reported that she had become withdrawn, preferred to stay in the home, and had been the subject of much peer rejection and teasing. The father was a passive individual who expressed resentment but was dependent upon his dominant wife, whom he viewed as more capable than himself.

Intellectual testing on more than one occasion revealed a full-scale IQ in the bright normal range. Neurological examination was within normal limits, but the EEG was reported as minimally abnormal with recurrent slow theta waves, five to seven per second, in right posterior areas and amplitude asymmetry, left occiput more than right occiput. This record was similar to one made about a month earlier except that the first record showed paroxysmal bursts.

Haloperidol was instituted in April, 1967, with good control of tics at a dosage of 2 mg of haloperidol twice daily. Over the next two years, dosage was adjusted between 4 mg and 16 mg of haloperidol daily. Symptoms were better controlled at higher doses, but side effects (blurred vision, lethargy, poor muscle coordination) were a problem, and benztropine mesylate, 1 mg twice daily, was used to help control them. With the addition of imipramine (Tofranil), 25 mg three times daily in 1968, the patient showed marked improvement, becoming more cheerful, alert, and less irritable and interacting more with other children. School work also improved.

When seen again in January, 1969, the patient showed frequent eye-blinking, but other tics were minimal. The mother reported that school grades and peer relations had deteriorated and that the patient "looked and acted stupid" at times. Dosage at this time was haloperidol, 12 mg daily, benztropine mesylate, 5 mg thrice daily, and imipramine, 25 mg thrice daily. Tics increased during the next three months, but increase of haloperidol to 16 mg daily gave little benefit. The mother undertook to stop medication for a time, but tics increased, and the patient became more excitable, irritable, and "brittle," so haloperidol was re-instituted at 14 mg daily. Since January, 1970, the patient has been under treatment at the Mayo Clinic in Minnesota. Here haloperidol was gradually decreased over a period of months to 6 mg daily at last report, and benztropine mesylate was discontinued. The mother reports that the patient is less sleepy but that blinking and screwing up of the eyes have increased.

Case 18

This boy (B.M., B.D. 7-22-54) was first seen at our clinic in 1964 at age 10 primarily because of a problem with motor tics and "noises," which had begun at age 7, but also because of behavioral problems. It was obvious that he was living in an extremely unhappy and unsatisfying household. The parents interacted hostilely, and the patient and his father were in constant conflict. The father was a rigid and strict individual, the mother more permissive and lenient toward the children. At the time of this first evaluation at the Child Psychiatry Service the patient received a full-scale IQ of 97. Neurological examination and EEG were essentially within normal limits, but visual-motor performance was suggestive of minimal brain damage. The patient said his tics were generally getting worse and that when he was engaged in conversation, the tics diminished, but when he was under pressure or not otherwise occupied, the tics increased. A trial of haloperidol was recommended to the referring source, but this was not carried out.

The patient was re-evaluated in October, 1968, at age 14 because of increasing behavioral problems in school relating to the motor tics and increased intensity and frequency of guttural noises. During interview, some throat-clearing sounds were noted, but no tics. However, when observed in the waiting room, both motor and vocal tics were much more obvious.

A trial of haloperidol was instituted with dosage gradually increased to 4 mg/day with an anti-Parkinsonism drug. The symptoms came under excellent control, and the patient and his parents reported that he was much more relaxed and showed no vocal or motor tics. On one occasion when the medication was lowered to 2 mg daily, the patient reported a return of some involuntary grunts and eye-blinking, which were controlled by returning the dosage to 4 mg daily.

Despite continued deterioration of the home situation, necessitating placement of the patient in a boarding school for a time, symptom control continued to be good through the last follow-up in 1970. In January, 1970, the patient said he could at times feel the symptoms breaking through, so dosage was increased to 6 mg of haloperidol daily along with 1 mg of benztropine mesylate twice daily. Some initial sleepiness appeared but passed off in about a week, and symptoms were again under complete control.

Case 19

This boy (R.L., B.D. 12-23-56) was first noticed to have tic-like symptoms (blinking of the eyes, facial and hand tics, and waving of the arms) in kindergarten, at about age 5. The symptoms progressed until his whole body became involved, and coprolalia developed at age 9 in 1965. A rather punitive teacher in the early grades exacerbated the symptoms because of her hysterical screaming. The patient's guardians, his aunt and uncle (who became his foster father and foster mother), tended at times to be punitive because they felt the patient could control his symptoms voluntarily. In 1965 the patient was placed in residential treatment for a 15-month period, and a psychiatrist from our clinic diagnosed Tourette's syndrome. Haloperidol was prescribed, and symptoms were almost completely controlled, at a dosage of 8 mg daily. The patient returned home to attend regular school. Three years later, at age 13, the medication was reduced by a local physician over a period of 4 weeks to no medication. Within two months, the motor tics, jerking of the head, and waving of the hands had returned. Because of the severity of the tics, the patient was completely exhausted while in the school situation and was allowed to leave school voluntarily a month later, when he was re-evaluated at our clinic. He displayed the symptoms noted above and poked his hands towards the interviewer's face and genital area. Haloperidol was re-instituted, the dosage being gradually raised to the previous dose of 8 mg daily. Antiparkinsonian drugs were also given. Initially there was good control at home, but when the patient returned to school, the pressures there exacerbated his tics, although they were less frequent. Medication was gradually raised over the next two months to a maximum of 20 mg haloperidol daily and benztropine mesylate, 1 mg twice daily. Each time medication was increased, symptoms were brought under partial and temporary control, only to return again apparently as a result of the increased pressure of school and home problems. When the patient was readmitted to our service in February, 1970 (age 14), he showed motor tics of the extremities as well as waving of the arms and some evidence of vocal tics, including very quiet coprolalia. Initially the patient's symptoms increased, but as he adjusted to the support of the new milieu and the less demanding school situation, the symptoms began to remit. First the coprolalia stopped, then vocal grunting ceased, and much of the excessive jerking of the head and shoulders abated. Because some organic brain dysfunction was suspected due to a mildly abnormal EEG, the patient was given a trial of first dextroamphetamine and then methylphenidate (Ritalin). On both occasions the symptoms became markedly worse during the 2 days of medication. Two months after rehospitalization, the patient's only symptoms were occasional motor tics, waving or poking of his hands towards eyes, ears, or genitals of personnel, and occasional obscene finger motions. Haloperidol had been gradually reduced from 20 mg daily to none. When off medication, the patient showed somewhat increased irritability and hostility toward the staff.

Case 20

This female patient (K.S., B.D. 10-15-60) was evaluated at our clinic in November, 1969, at age 9. Symptoms first began in kindergarten with jerking of the head and clearing of the throat. The patient was also described as being very overactive and distractable in the classroom. The teacher was quite annoyed about the child's behavior and called the stepmother on the average once daily. The tics progressed to include jerking of the head and shoulders and guttural tics and noises which progressed to coprolalia. In 1967 (age 7) the patient was transferred to a special school for learning disabilities and here, under reduced stress and the greater tolerance of the teachers, symptoms became much less pronounced. In June, 1969, the vocal tics, particularly coprolalia, returned. To punish this, the parents washed the patient's mouth out with soap for the first few weeks three times daily. When the patient returned to her special school in the fall of 1969, the principal refused to tolerate her verbal tics and took a punitive attitude which exacerbated her symptoms and finally led to her being excluded from school.

When evaluated at our clinic in November, 1969, the patient's error score on the Bender Gestalt was more than 5 deviations above her age, evidencing a serious visual-motor problem. The neurological examination was well within normal limits except for slight awkwardness of gait. Previous psychological testing revealed a full-scale WISC IQ of 85 with wide variability in individual scale scores, ranging from a low of 5 on the arithmetic subtest to a high of 11 on the information subtest. This was thought to be a very low estimate of the child's potential in view of her extreme distractability and short attention span.

The patient was friendly, interested, and very cooperative, but obviously overactive. Throughout the interview she used many coprolalic words and there were other vocal tics and unintelligible utterances. When the patient was left alone, coprolalia decreased markedly, but the vocal tics and barking noises increased considerably, to about one every 4 or 5 seconds. Haloperidol was instituted, and as dosage was gradually raised symptoms decreased to a symptom-free point at 2 mg haloperidol daily, and she was described by her teacher, parents, and others as "a new child." Notwithstanding this, the principal of the special school refused to readmit her, but she was fortunately accepted in the regular third grade in January, 1970. The patient remained overactive at times, but displayed none of the symptoms of Tourette's syndrome, integrated well into the class, and made reasonable scholastic progress. Minor coprolalia (soft, almost unintelligible) broke through occasionally, but increase in medication to 2 mg twice daily quickly controlled the symptoms once again. Because of the child's hyperkinetic symptoms, a 5-day trial of dextroamphetamine was undertaken, 15 mg in a long-acting release form each morning. The patient seemed somewhat less hyperkinetic and distractable, but vocal tics returned and caused the school some concern. When dextroamphetamine was discontinued, symptoms abated, and the patient was well controlled on haloperidol 3 mg twice daily.

Case 21 — Comparison case

This female patient (D.M.) was referred to our clinic in January, 1970, with a diagnostic impression of Tourette's disease. We do not now believe that this impression was correct, but present the case for comparison purposes. The diagnosis of Tourette's syndrome had been made by a mental health center in 1968 on the basis of coprolalia (such as "fuck," usually shouted at times of stress). The parents did not recall the usual progression of Tourette's symptoms such as blinking of the eyes or facial or other motor tics gradually involving the entire body, nor did throat-clearing or guttural noises precede the coprolalia. The patient was placed on 3 mg haloperidol daily, and coprolalia disappeared entirely and has not reappeared. Because of "sassy, defiant behavior," especially toward her mother, the patient was placed in a county home, enrolled in a nearby school for emotionally disturbed children, and medication was increased to 5 mg haloperidol daily plus 150 mg chlorpromazine daily, the latter the usual county home dose given to virtually all inmates. The patient presented no behavior problems either at the home or in school.

At our evaluation in 1970, the patient appeared as a quiet, cooperative, poorly groomed, shy, and obviously immature girl of borderline intelligence who was obviously extremely sleepy and under excessive sedation. Neurological examination and visual motor tests were within normal limits. The patient was hospitalized while medication was gradually reduced from 5 mg daily to none over a period of 3 weeks. No symptoms of Tourette's syndrome appeared during that time or since. Follow-up is being continued to see whether the original diagnosis was indeed in error.

SECTION TWO: CURRENT INVESTIGATIONS

Contributions to the International Registry

Gilles de la Tourette's Syndrome. Volume 1: International Registry, p. 71-79, edited by F. Abuzzahab Sr. and F. Anderson. Mason Publishing Co., St. Paul ©1976.

GILLES DE LA TOURETTE'S SYNDROME: CROSS-CULTURAL ANALYSIS AND TREATMENT OUTCOME

F. S. Abuzzahab Sr., M.D., Ph.D.
Clinical Associate Professor
Departments of Psychiatry, Pharmacology and Family Practice and Community Health
University of Minnesota
Minneapolis, Minnesota 55455 U.S.A.

and

Floyd O. Anderson, M.D.
Resident in Psychiatry
University of Minnesota
Minneapolis, Minnesota 55455 U.S.A.

The syndrome of Gilles de la Tourette, with its peculiar motor and vocal symptomatology, has fascinated medical professionals all over the world. Its etiology is obscure even after over a hundred years of observations, and only recently have its symptoms been controllable. In order to obtain case reports of the illness, an exhaustive search of the literature was conducted, and an international registry was set up. This report is based upon information pooled from the first 430 case reports in our files.

An empirical description of the syndrome's natural history has been assembled. Symptomatology as well as certain informative aspects will be described. These characteristics will then be analyzed cross-culturally between the five statistically significant groups, based on national origin. Finally, the results of the various therapies which have been tried on Tourette tiqueurs over the years will be compared.

HISTORY

The first description of the syndrome, albeit sketchy, was in 1810 by Bouteille[56] in his "Treatise on Chorea." Itard[232] presented the case report in 1825 of the Marquise de Dampierre, then 26 years old. This influential woman had developed the symptoms of Tourette's syndrome at the age of 7 and, because of coprolalia and echolalia, spent most of her long life in seclusion.

Her case was to be the classic case of Tourette's syndrome. It was reported by Roth in 1850 and again by Sandras in 1851, by Trousseau in 1873, who called it "diaphragmatic chorea", and by H. Jones in 1874. She was seen by Gilles de la Tourette, Charcot, and Mirto at the Salpetriere in the early 1880's, and her case was mentioned in Gilles de la Tourette's 1885 analysis of nine cases entitled "A Nervous Affection Characterized by Motor Incoordination, Accompanied by Echolalia and Coprolalia."[198]

All of the early work was not done by the French, however. In 1881 (four years before Tourette's description), Friedreich published a case report of what he called "Koordinierte Erinnerungskrampfe", which was identical with the syndrome of Gilles de la Tourette.[182]

Gilles de la Tourette, prior to 1885, had taken interest in Beard's work of 1880 on the "jumpers" of Maine, O'Brien's report on "latah" in Malaya and Hammond's treatise on "myriachit" in Siberia. This led to his 1884 paper[197] which collected previous observations and reported one of his own. He felt that these various illnesses were in fact the same. He reasserted this opinion in his classic paper of 1885, which proved his ability as a gifted observer and nosologist; thus the syndrome was named after him.

Some of the most significant work since 1885 includes:

1890: Jacques Catrou, another student of Charcot at the Salpêtrière, presented a detailed history and 45 case summaries in his inaugural dissertation.[80]

1899: Koester found 50 cases in a review of the literature, and presented the two cases of Tourette's syndrome diagnosed in 2500 admissions at the

Universitats Poliklinik in Leipzig.[255]
1946: Mahler reports a series of 10 patients studied from one to eleven years.[300]
1948: Eduard Ascher finds 4 cases among 9000 inpatient and 50,000 outpatient admissions to a psychiatric clinic.[11]
1961: Seignot successfully treats Gilles de la Tourette's syndrome with haloperidol.[415]
1961: Salmi finds one case of the syndrome among 5300 children at the Education Guidance Clinic in Finland.[401]
1966: Feild, *et al*, report on 7 cases diagnosed out of 1.5 million admissions to the Mayo Clinic since 1935.[162]
1967: Challas and co-workers analyze 57 case reports in a review of the literature since 1942.[85]
1970: Snyder compares various therapies in 108 cases of Gilles de la Tourette's syndrome.[430]

SUMMARY OF CASE REPORTS

Tourette's syndrome has been known variously as **maladie de tics,**[81] **tic convulsif,**[207] **tic impulsif,**[488] **mimische Krampfneurose,**[62] and other names. Since it is typically variable in its clinical presentation, the empirical description that follows may be helpful to the clinician. The following data reflect the symptoms and historical picture evidence at clinical presentation.

FIGURE I

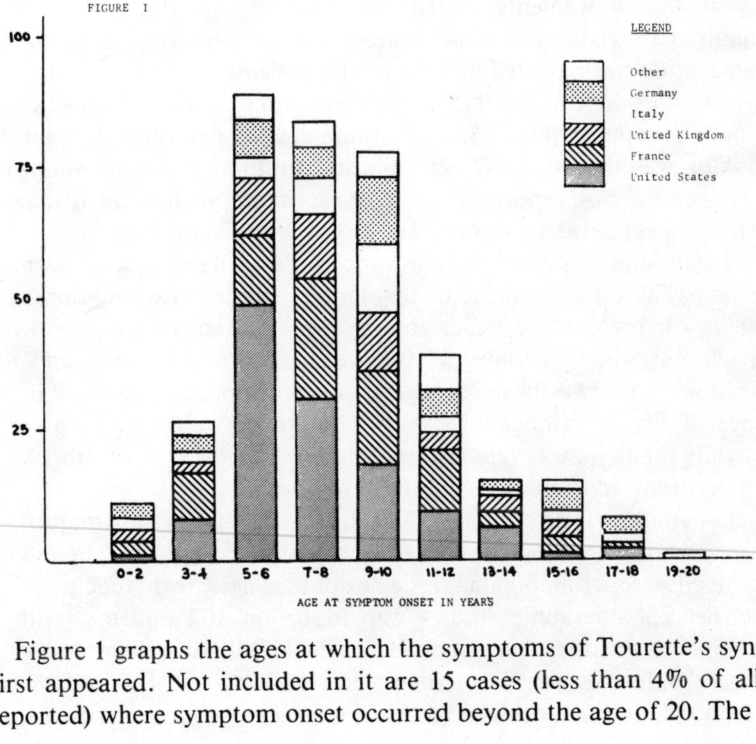

Figure 1 graphs the ages at which the symptoms of Tourette's syndrome first appeared. Not included in it are 15 cases (less than 4% of all cases reported) where symptom onset occurred beyond the age of 20. The age of onset in fully 90% of reported cases was between 3 and 16 years, with over three-fourths between the ages of 5 and 12 years.

Seventy-one percent of Tourette-tiqueurs are males, although the classic patient was a woman, first described by Itard in 1825 and by four other authors, including Gilles de la Tourette himself, in the next 65 years. The frequencies of symptoms are presented in Table I. Motor symptoms include

TABLE I: FREQUENCY OF SYMPTOMS

Motor Symptoms:	
Facial tics	92%
Arm tics	78%
Leg tics	54%
Neck tics	53%
Eye tics	31%
Vocal Symptoms:	
Inarticulations	65%
Coprolalia	58%
Echolalia	23%

mainly tic-like movements, often coordinated and fluctuating. Most commonly the facial mimic muscles are involved: grimacing, blinking and other facial tics are reported in 92% of the patients. Arm tics occurred in 78%, while only 54% had gait disturbance or frank leg tics. Head jerks and other neck tics appeared in 53% and, although several authors thought that eyeblinking was the most frequent motor symptom, it was mentioned in only 31% of the case reports. Involuntary imitation of movements, called echopraxia or echokinesis, was present in only 9% of these cases.

Vocal symptoms reported include various inarticulations, such as barks and monosyllables; coprolalia, or involuntary obscene exclamations; and echolalia, or involuntary repetition of the spoken or written word. Inarticulations were generally the first vocalizations to appear, and they were reported in two-thirds of the patients. Coprolalia, which in the presence of tics is pathognomonic of Tourette's syndrome, occurred in 58%, while echolalia was reported in only one-fourth. One or more vocal symptoms occurred in over 90% of the patients.

Psychopathology was present in 33% of the cases. The vast majority of these were various neuroses classified as obsessive-compulsive. Frequently encountered were arithmomania, folie de doute and delire du touche.

Electroencephalographic studies were done on 102 patients, with 45 producing abnormal results. Figure II depicts the distribution of scores on the Wechsler Intelligence Scale for Children. Forty-five full scale scores were reported, with almost normal distribution except for a preponderance

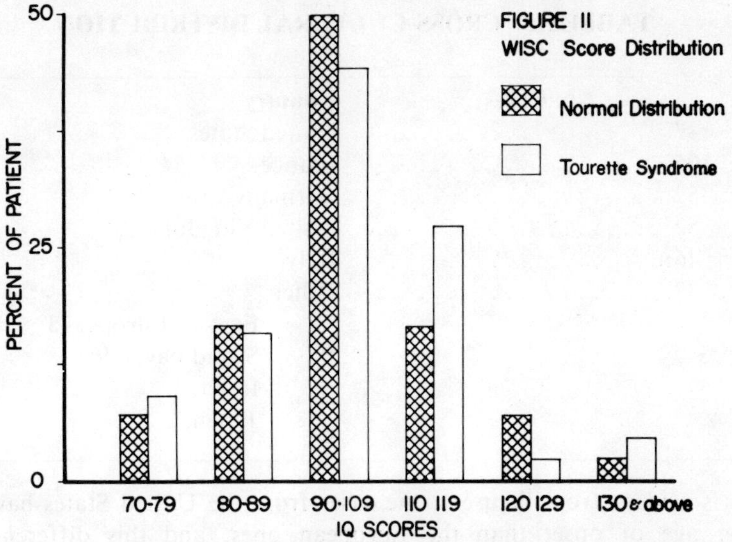

of scores in the 110-119 range. In 66 case reports, intelligence was described as "average", with 26 "above average" and 14 "below average."

A family history of neuroticism was found in 57%, but this figure is misleading since positive findings were of common and unrelated problems, and rarely was there any extrapyramidal tract involvment. Only in three cases was another family member a Tourette tiqueur.

Among the many possible causes that have been suggested for Tourette's syndrome are birth damage, early traumatic events or infectious diseases, and family dynamics. Birth abnormalities and abnormal growth and development were reported in only 15% of patients, and none of these were frequent enough to indicate any connection with the development of the illness. On the other hand, a precipitating event was described in 161 cases or 37%. Most frequently associated with symptom onset were infections and various traumatic episodes, with no significant incidence of encephalitis or probable encephalitis (3%).

There is evidence that family dynamics may be a contributing factor if one or both parents are strict or dominating, or if the domestic situation is in other ways hostile. This was the case with 135 patients, which is significant when given the fact that such data were seldom reported by early investigators.

Cross Cultural Analysis

When the 430 cases were divided into groups reflecting their national origin, as is seen in Table II, there were five groups (from the United States, France, the United Kingdom, Italy and Germany) with a sufficient number of patients so that significant statistical comparisons could be made. Each group was analyzed against all cases not in that group by the Chi Square method. (Graph in Figure 1).

TABLE II: CROSS-CULTURAL DISTRIBUTION

No. Cases	Country
137	United States
105	France
57	Germany
52	United Kingdom
46	Italy
33	Other: Eastern Europe, 13; Scandinavia, 9; India, 5; Japan, 2

As is evident from Figure 1, the cases from the United States have an earlier age of onset than the European ones, and this difference is statistically significant.

There were few significant deviations in motor symptoms between groups and the male-female ratio also showed an excellent fit. The high correlations between samples in all but a few instances were impressive. However, the Italian sample showed a significantly higher frequency of eye tics, while the French showed significantly fewer. More neck tics were observed in the United States sample, and fewer in the French.

A similarly close fit was not found with the copro- and echo-phenomena, however. The British group displayed significantly less echophenomena, while the other vocal phenomena fit closely. On the other hand, the French group showed much more echokinesis than expected. Many of the patients in earlier reports from France presented this symptom, which was described in the French literature of the early 1880's. Perhaps the novelty of this fascinating symptom led to its frequent diagnosis.

Coprolalia was found to occur in the United States with a significantly higher frequency than elsewhere, although other vocal symptoms occurred with expected frequencies. Despite the many statistically significant differences found in other groups, the German sample corresponded very well and could be described as the typical group.

Results of Therapy

Table III gives the results of the most frequently used modes of treatment. In the 430 cases of the study, there were just 600 therapeutic trials, many patients being given more than one type of treatment.

Different types of psychotherapy were frequently employed with Gilles de la Tourette's patients. Forty-five percent were described as "improved", but only 12% for more than six months. Behavioral modification therapy produced six-month "improvement" in 25% of trials, but had a 75% failure rate.

TABLE III

Comparative Efficacy of Various Treatments in Gilles de la Tourette's Syndrome

Treatment	No. of Patient Trials	Treatment Failures	Improvement of Unknown Duration	Improvement for less than 6 mos.	Improvement for more than 6 mos.	% Improved for more than 6 mos.	Total % Improved
Psychotherapy	117	65	31	7	14	12	45
Hypnotherapy	27	23	2	0	2	7	15
Hydrotherapy	25	22	1	2	0	0	12
Isolation	19	14	0	3	2	11	26
Sleep therapy	13	6	4	3	0	0	54
Behavior therapy	12	9	0	0	3	25	25
Bed rest	6	4	1	1	0	0	33
Shock therapy	25	20	3	2	0	0	20
CO_2 Inhalation	11	9	o	1	1	9	18
Physical therapy	9	4	4	1	0	0	56
Thalamotomy	3	2	0	0	1	33	33
Lobotomy-leucotomy	2	1	0	0	1	50	50
Sedatives[1]	98	79	11	4	4	4	19
Antipsychotic Tranq[2]	81	42	16	5	18	22	48
Haloperidol	63	7	8	6	42	67	89
Antidepressants[3]	17	13	1	3	0	0	24
CNS stimulants[4]	17	14	1	1	1	6	18
Anticonvulsants[5]	16	13	2	0	1	6	19
Antiparkinsonians[6]	7	5	0	1	1	14	29
Spontaneous Remission	14	(representing 3.3% of patients)					

Analysis of various therapies reported in 430 case histories of Gilles de la Tourette's syndrome surveyed in the literature (often several therapeutic trials were given to the same patient). (1) "Sedatives": ethanol, chloral hydrate, ethchlorvynol, bromides, barbiturates, meprobamate, chlordiazepoxide, diazepam, oxazepam, hydroxyzine, methaqualone, arsenic, paraldehyde. (2) "Anti-psychotic tranquilizers": reserpine, rauwolfia alkaloids, chlorpromazine, promazine, triflupromazine, thioridazine, prochlorperazine, trifluperazine, chlorprothixene, fluphenazine, perphenazine, thiothixene, piperacetazine, promethazine. (3) "antidepressants": imipramine, amitriptyline, nortriptyline, doxepin, protriptyline, isocarboxazid, phenelzine, iproniazid. (4) "CNS stimulants": amphetamine, d-amphetamine, methamphetamine, methylphenidate. (5) "Anticonvulsants": diphenylhydantoin, primadone, trimethadione, ethosuximide, paramethadione. (6) "Anti-parkinsonians": belladonna alkaloids, trihexyphenidyl, benztropine mesylate, orphenadrine, diphenhydramine, L-dopa, amantadine.

The results of chemotherapy are difficult to evaluate due to the simultaneous administration of different classes of drugs. However, the benefit of haloperidol is plain. Fully two-thirds of its therapeutic trials gave a greater than six-month "improvement", and 89% of trials produced some "improvement". The other anti-psychotic tranquilizers produced "improvement" in 48% of trials, with 22% giving long-term "improvement".

Other modes of therapy not tabulated, many of them now known to be undesirable, do not seem to be valuable in the control of Tourette symptoms. These miscellaneous therapies include chiropractic treatment, lysergic acid diethylamide (LSD), fever therapy, hygiene, flogging, strictness, megavitamins, leeches and muscle relaxants.

It is of note that 14 patients (3.3%) had spontaneous remissions at 6-month follow-up.

DISCUSSION

Over two-thirds (71%) of Tourette patients in our sample were males, comparing closely to the ratios observed by Gilles de la Tourette and subsequent investigators. A similar preponderance of males is seen with simple tics. The key clinical features leading to the diagnosis of Tourette's syndrome in this study were childhood onset (90.5% between 3 and 16 years) of more or less generalized motor tics involving most frequently the face (98%) and the upper extremities (78%). One or more vocal symptoms, either inarticulations, coprolalia or echolalia, were present in 93% of cases at some time during the course of the illness. In the vast majority of cases, the vocal symptoms led to the diagnosis, although coprolalia, considered pathognomonic of the syndrome, occurred in just 65% of the cases.

The syndrome's course is typified by remissions and exacerbations with fluctuating symptomatology. Spontaneous remissions of six months or more were observed in only 14 reported cases (3.3%).

There are no diagnostic tests of value currently. However, Messiha, *et al*[319] report that levels of urinary catecholamines, notably dopamine, fluctuated directly with the severity of symptoms in a patient with Tourette's syndrome. Earlier, Snyder, *et al* [430] hypothesized that hypersecretion of dopamine in the corpus striatum could be at least part of the pathophysiological picture, given the startling improvement seen with haloperidol therapy.

The cross-cultural comparison of case histories showed that the main features of the syndrome are similar, with some variation in symptom expression as summarized in Table IV.

TABLE IV: CROSS-CULTURAL SYMPTOM DIFFERENCES*

United States:	Younger age at onset More neck tics More coprolalia
France:	Less neck tics Less eye tics More echokinesis
Germany:	No significant differences
United Kingdom:	Less echophenomena
Italy:	More eye tics

* Using the Chi-squared method with $P < 0.05$.

The statistically significant variation in symptom expression could represent the bias of authors from particular cultural settings. One difficulty in our attempts at cross-cultural analysis was that only 33 cases (7.7%) were reported from countries other than the United States, France, the United Kingdom, Italy and Germany, most of the others being Eastern European. The higher incidence of case reports from the Western nations may reflect eagerness to publish rather than an actual higher incidence of the illness.

The comparison of different treatment regimes used with these patients shows that haloperidol is superior to any other treatment, and must be considered the treatment of choice in Gilles de la Tourette's syndrome. The anti-psychotic tranquilizers have some value, but the efficacy of psychotherapy and other regimes is questionable.

In order to more fully understand the natural history of this disorder and to elucidate the exact role of haloperidol in attenuating its symptoms, an international registry has been founded. Physicians are encouraged to contribute their clinical observations to this registry by contributing to the senior author of this article.

Gilles de la Tourette's Syndrome. Volume 1: International Registry, p. 81-87, edited by F. Abuzzahab Sr. and F. Anderson. Mason Publishing Co., St. Paul ©1976.

GILLES DE LA TOURETTE'S DISEASE WITH CONGENITAL VASCULAR MALFORMATIONS AND SECONDARY ENCEPHALOPATHY

Wlodzimierz Borak, M.D.
Hospital for Nervous Diseases
Gniezno, Poland

and

Ewa Osetowska, M.D.
Institute of Comparative Neuropathology
Centre of Experimental and Clinical Medicine
Polish Academy of Sciences
Gniezno, Poland

In 1940, Wilson pointed to the decreasing incidence of Gilles de la Tourette's disease. In support of his statement he wrote, ". . . I can find no case report in recent times. Twenty-five years ago a typical example came under my personal notice". The situation seems to have changed in the past twenty years. This interesting syndrome, which is characterized by the progressive development of multiple tics, echo- and coprolalia, echokinesis and compulsive acts, has relatively frequently been observed by Polish psychiatrists also.[142]

Compared with clinical descriptions, neuropathological findings have less frequently been published. The picture of the brain is usually non-characteristic, as can be seen from the descriptions of Clauss and Balthazar.[97 18] This is probably why the etiology of Gilles de la Tourette's disease is still controversial. Some authors feel it is brought about by psychogenic factors.[442 153 324 426 441] Others have always thought it to be of organic origin, inflammatory,[38] posttraumatic,[293] or hypoplastic.[97] The idea of a third group is that Gilles de la Tourette's disease is attributable to psychogenic stratification in individuals with organic brain damage. The latter view is represented in literature by van Bogaert,[460] and the Bilikiewicz school in Poland.[37]

The reason for these differences of view is presumably the fact that the functional component of this syndrome is not always easy to distinguish from the organic. Surgical intervention in the case described here allowed a certain differentiation of symptoms. The case was first published in Poland[52] during the patient's lifetime. A comprehensive picture is now presented, including postoperative course and neuropathological examination.

Case Report

M.Z., 9 years old, was admitted to our hospital on September 4, 1960. According to the history he was the child of unknown parents and had been adopted by a foster family. In his second year he began to walk, but did not speak until his fourth year. Since the age of three, he would often strike his head with his hands. At the age of four he went through a febrile illness with irritation of the cerebrospinal meninges and, in the initial stage, disorders of consciousness. There was suspicion of typhoid fever.

Neurological examinations performed after admission revealed tremor of the tongue and very brisk deep reflexes, as well as a number of tic-like movements becoming more intense under the influence of emotional stimuli. He would squint his eyes, lift his eyebrows, open his mouth wide, put out his tongue, grind his teeth, inhale air deeply, suddenly spit at his entourage, and perform rhythmic tremor-like movements with his upper extremities. He uttered single vowels or syllables, unable to restrain himself from doing so for more than 10-15 seconds. He also uttered vulgar words, although more rarely.

He had a very short attention span and an inclination to monologizing; a conversation of a few minutes made him yawn. His interest was restricted to merely physiological needs and trifling topics of which he spoke continually in a stereotyped manner, expressing endless doubts and fears.

Test examinations with the Binet-Termann scale revealed mental retardation of about 2 years.

The child was usually very cheerful, often too much so, considering the situation, but he often changed his mood and became obstinate and insolent. A nurse observed that he would stamp his feet, tear his pajamas into pieces, and bang a chair on the floor. When irritated, he would strike his head with his fists or bang it against the wall. He was constantly in motion. At school, he was unable to do any work unless the teacher was standing by him. He was unable to play with other children, nor did he want to. His face had a dull expression, and his voice was monotonous and poorly modulated. He was deeply attached to his foster mother.

Ancillary routine examinations revealed no abnormalities. An electroencephalogram performed on March 10, 1960, gave an abnormal record, with generalized cerebral changes of the medium degree; the left hemisphere was slightly larger than the right. Another encephalogram on September 22, 1966, gave a record within the limits of normal. Air encephalography on December 19, 1963 revealed marked hydrocephalic dilatation of the left lateral ventricle. The right ventricle was not dilated, but showed rounding of the upper lateral cornu. The third ventricle was slightly dilated.

The boy's condition became much worse in the fifth week after admission. Mild febrile episodes were observed. The second sound over the pulmonary artery was accentuated. Blood sedimentation was increased, to a maximum of 50 mm per hr. Neurological examinations revealed hyperactive deep tendon reflexes and hypoactive abdominal reflexes on the left side. Slight central paresis of the right facial nerve was discovered.

Motor tics continued with still greater intensity; several new tics developed. The boy would bite on his lips and tongue, perform semicircular rocking-like left to right neck movements and rapid nodding movements, and thrust his mandible forward. Coprolalia and other verbal tics became more intense. The frequency of masturbation and spitting-type tics was also increased. Self-aggression was markedly potentiated owing to motor tics consisting of sudden, very rapid flexing of the elbow joints. At first, the boy was able to control these phenomena, holding his hands down himself or asking for help. After a time, however, if his hands were not held down, he would bend not only the elbow but also the carpal joints, compress his fist and strike a hard blow, usually at his head. His lower extremities were less involved, although, if they were not held down, he would bend both knee and hip joints and hit his head with his knees. These movements were less violent when his extremities were immobilized. Were this not done, as he himself wished, he might have killed himself.

All these phenomena were associated with anxiety and innumerable doubts and ponderings. The boy was in deadly fear that the nurses might fail to hold his hands down. He would strike the people around him, bang his head against the wall, and cry and shriek frequently. A dysphoric mood prevailed.

Blood sedimentation returned to normal (14 mm per hr.) in the course of anti-rheumatic treatment administered in the third month of his stay in the hospital. The febrile states receded after a year.

The patient received treatment with chlorpromazine (maximum daily dose 300 mg), thioridazine (150 mg/day), phenobarbital (200 mg/day) and haloperidol (9 mg/day). Slight improvement consisting of a reduction in tic intensity was attained in the course of each of these treatments, without, however, reaching the tics associated with self-aggression. Relapses were observed in the course of somatic illnesses, particularly following influenza.

In 1969, the patient underwent surgery in the department of neurosurgery of the Polish Academy of Sciences (Dr. Mempel). Left cryothalamotomy, performed on May 5, 1969, produced no improvement; involuntary face movements and tendencies toward self-aggression continued. Right cryothalamotomy was performed on May 22, 1969. On may 25, 1969 there were fewer face tics but tendencies toward self-aggression remained unchanged. On June 8, there were fewer involuntary movements. He began to walk.

After readmission to our hospital he suffered more frequently from dysphoria. States of psychomotor agitation became more and more intense appearing daily and lasting for hours in spite of barbiturates and neuroleptics. The boy would then become quite uninhibited. Although his extremities and chest were immobilized, and his knees and shoulders protected, he tossed his body about, uttering loud shrieks and displaying motor tics and coprolalia. Face tics were seldom observed. Febrile states continued despite a normal physical examination. Exacerbation was observed during a heatwave.

The patient died on July 27, 1969 because of circulatory insufficiency.

Anatomopathological diagnosis

The brain, fixed in 10% formalin, was symmetrical, with meningeal vessels congested, sulci obliterated, and meninges near the interhemispherical fissure slightly milky. On the fronto-paracentral borderline were two symmetrical postoperative lesions. On the transverse section were found some small foci of demyelination in the white matter of the centrum semiovale. Brain stem and cerebellem showed macroscopic changes.

Microscopic technique

Sections through the hemispheres from the frontal, paracentral and parieto-occipital levels bilaterally, and from the pons, mesencephalon, the medulla, and both cerebellar hemispheres were embedded in paraffin blocks and stained by the following methods: Nissl, Heidenhain, van Gieson and hematoxylin-eosin.

Microscopic examination

Cortex: The frontal, paracentral, parietal, temporal and occipital areas showed extensive neuronal deficits disturbing the normal cortical layers.

There was a relationship evident between the loss of neurons and proximity to the altered vessels. The preserved nerve cells showed various alterations ranging from faint staining to severe and ischemic degeneration. The rarefactions in the small-cell cortical layers were partly covered with proliferated glial nuclei. The large Betz cells in the pyramidal layer were rarefied and altered. Cortical vessels were surrounded by extensive transudates with sporadic intratissular spongiform foci.

The white matter: The subcortical areas showed vessels with disintegrated walls surrounded by minute hemorrhages, with proliferating microglia (Fig. 1). There was, besides, a strikingly large number of underdeveloped, thin-

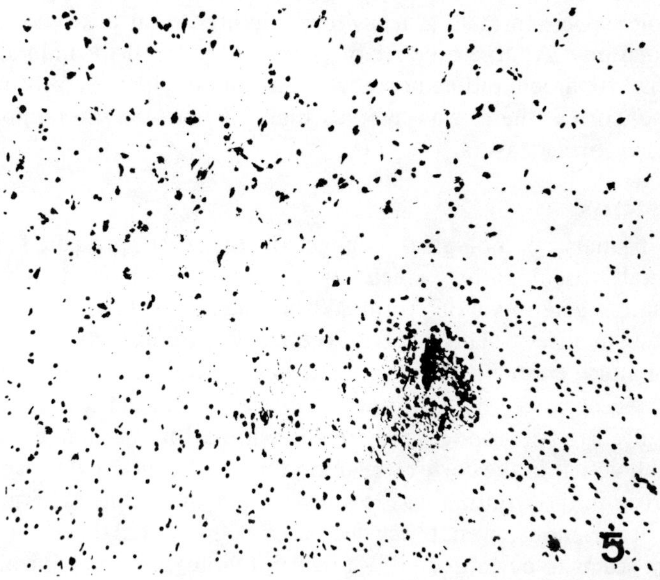

Figure 1. Disintegrating vessel with minute hemorrhage and microglial reaction in the subcortical white matter. Paraffin, cresol-violet stain, x150.

walled vessels, as well as vessels secondarily degenerated, with hyaloid or fibrous changes and intimal proliferation. The foci of postoperative lesions found in the vicinity of these vascular groups showed a very rich fibroblastic organization with posthemorrhagic lacunae in the center, and calcium deposits. Diffuse demyelination near the postoperative lesions and around larger vessels corresponded to edematous areas, and cell staining revealed an irregular pattern of oligodendroglial nuclei.

Basal ganglia: A large number of vessels surrounded by edematous halos were found in the thalamus, the striatum and the pallidum. The transudate expanding from the perivascular spaces involved the nerve cells, causing lesions similar to those observed in the cortex. Where larger vessels were concerned, the picture resembled early phases of status lacunaris. The walls of a good number of striatal vessels showed a deficient transitory arteriovenous structure. Large and small neurons in the vicinity of the altered vessels appeared damaged. The intrastriatal fibers were swollen and slightly demyelinated. There were postoperative scars, rather small and mostly glial, in the two latero-ventral nuclei of the thalamus.

Brain stem and cerebellum: Nerve cell rarefactions within the substantia nigra, the cranial nerve nuclei and the olives were, in the vicinity of the changed vessels, similar to those occurring at higher levels. The cerebellar white matter showed perivascular loss in the cerebellar granular layer and deficits in the Purkinje cells, as well as large lacunae around the arterial and venous vessels.

Some of the numerous atypical arteries and veins lying in the subarachnoid space formed a transitory picture of arteriovenous racemic malformations. A large number of them had parietal thrombi alternating with small subarachnoid hemorrhages. Around the large vessels proceeding into the cortex there was perivascular edematous rarefaction in the superficial cortical layers.

DISCUSSION

The primary pathological change in the case presented here was congenital vasculopathy which at the meningeal level assumed an angiomatous arterio-venous form. Within the cerebral tissue, these changes were less manifest. There were secondary vascular changes, some of inflammatory character with a tendency toward intimal proliferation, others degenerative, as hyalinosis, fibrosis and calcification. Neuronal lesions occurred in topographic relationship with vascular changes. The nerve cell deficit in the cortex was undoubtedly the most extensive. The loss of neurons in the striatum was less severe, but the cellular alterations were always conspicuous, even if they decreased in the caudal direction.

There seems to be conformity of neuropathological and clinical features. The syndrome of mental retardation, together with mental disorders, may correspond to the disturbed brain metabolism caused by increased permeability of the blood-brain barrier. The disorders of a hemo-dynamic nature were increased by the inflammatory and infectious incidents revealed in the history (typhoid fever(?), measles, influenza, etc.), thus enhancing the loss of neurons in the vicinity of the vessels as well as the perivascular myelin breakdown.[460] The hypothesis of rheumatic encephalitis seems doubtful. Changes in the cortical vessels were slightly reminiscent of Bruetsch's rheumatic encephalopathy,[70] although they were far from presenting the rich picture of typical rheumatic encephalitis.[354] Of the greatest importance was the lack of cardiac rheumatic lesions which are essential for diagnosing rheumatic encephalopathy or encephalitis.[70] However, in a primary defective vascular system, the recurrence of common generalized infectious illnesses was sufficient to produce the parenchymal changes described. Under these conditions, the post-operative shock was particularly traumatic: this is demonstrated by the extensive cicatrizing proliferation.

The neuropathological findings also seem to point to Gilles de la Tourette's disease. Both Wilson[489] and van Bogaert[461] emphasized the complex character of motor disturbances in Gilles de la Tourette's syndrome. They thought "tics" to be at the borderline between involuntary movements in the organic sense and psychogenic compulsory motor disturbances. Consequently, Gilles de la Tourette's disease has at its base no systematic lesions involving selected cellular elements. In the case here presented, the neuropathological picture includes organic possibilities as well as psychic. The discharges of compulsory and emotional nature may have alternated with involuntary movements caused by organic cellular lesions. The simultaneous presence of an organic coefficient may have been an explanation for the transient improvement which had followed surgical intervention.

Gilles de la Tourette's Syndrome. Volume 1: International Registry, p. 89-98, edited by F. Abuzzahab Sr. and F. Anderson. Mason Publishing Co., St. Paul ©1976.

GILLES DE LA TOURETTE'S DISEASE

Marie Fisarova, C.Sc.
Department of Neurology
Husova 370
Strakonice, Czechoslovakia 386 01

In the year 1885, incited by his teacher Charcot, Gilles de la Tourette separated a special clinical unit from chorea and hysteria. Even if it is a relatively rare disease, it is still paid great attention by both neurologists and psychiatrists, the views on its etiology and prognosis being very different. We have been following 18 patients with this diagnosis for a long period of time and thus our experiences may contribute to the clarification of some literary disputes.

Case Reports

1. V.J., boy, born 1953. His grandfather committed suicide and his grandmother from the paternal side suffered from some kind of paroxysms. During pregnancy his mother had pains in the back, and in the seventh month of pregnancy she fell down from a carriage. The delivery was precipitated, the delivery weight of the child was 3.5 kg.

The boy started to sit at the age of 18 months, to walk at the age of four years. In the third month of life he suffered from pneumonia and diarrhea, was hospitalized for five weeks at the Department of Pediatrics and was sent home in a moribund condition. He was very often ill, had measles, frequent tonsillitis, otitis, whooping cough and mumps. He was restless and at the age of six abnormal blinking of his eyes started. Up to eight years of age he wet his bed.

At nine years the choreatic restlessness worsened. Spasmodic movements of the head occurred with brisk movements of the limbs, opening of mouth, snorting, frequent clearing of throat, producing sounds very similar to dog's barking. The psychomotor restlessness prevented his attending school. Repeatedly hospitalized at the Department of Neurology or Pediatrics, the X-ray picture of the skull, PEG, fundus and the pediatric findings were normal.

The EEG revealed slightly diffuse disturbances of electric activity and suggested an early-originated lesion of the stem structures. The curve corresponded to the perinatal lesion and did not exclude superimposed inflammatory or degenerative lesions. Spinal fluid at the very start of the disease revealed a protein level of 148 mg%, Pandy +, sugar 78 mg%, chlorides 760 mg%, with 16 lymphocytes and 21 PMN. Electrophoresis of spinal fluid showed albumins 71.5%, globulins: alpha/1 10%, alpha/2 7.2%, beta 7.2%, gamma 4.1%, A/G 2.51.

The control examination performed after 7 years revealed PEG proved atrophy of the cerebellum, as well as spinal fluid values: proteins 10 mg%, Pandy neg., sugar 65 mg%, chlorides 420 mg%. Electrophoresis of the fluid showed albumins 55.8%, globulins 42%, A/G 1.38. The EEG conclusively proved diffuse disturbance of electric activity with the signs of the stem lesion, which agrees with the presupposition of a degenerative disease on the perinatally damaged tissue.

The neurological findings up to the age of 3 years spoke for the extrapyramidal form of cerebral palsy. At age 8, muscular hypotonia, walking with a wide base, and choreo-athetoid movements were still present. At the age of 12, he exhibited dysplastic habitus, generalized tics, general muscular hypotrophy, and expressive atrophy of the muscles of both calves. Deep tendon reflexes were not evokable and Babinskis were positive bilaterally. He walked with a wide base and showed severe thoracic kyphoscoliosis. There was decreased sensitivity, both deep and superficial, on the lower extremities. Muscular biopsy did not reveal pathological changes. Electromyography spoke for a mixed lesion with the preponderance of the nuclear type, without any signs of a myogenic lesion.

The boy was a very bad pupil, his school attendance being interrupted by frequent hospitalizations. In spite of that, he finished school normally. The psychomotor restlessness and generalized tics of various intensity are still present, with echo- and coprolalia occurring from time to time. The boy rides a bicycle, plays ice hockey, and now works as a manual laborer. Tics are worse after any infectious disease, sometimes even after emotion.

The recent neurological findings speak for spinocerebellar degeneration of Friedreich's type, with preponderance of the dorsal and lateral medullary columns, with less expressed cerebellar symptomatology.

This case is the most remarkable in our series as it has been observed in detail since the patient was three months old. He was a perinatally lesioned infant, tics appearing at the pre-school age. At nine years, the findings corresponded to Gilles de la Tourette's disease, and now the spinocerebellar degeneration comes to the fore in addition to the previous findings. Cerebrospinal fluid examinations at the very start of the disease proved an inflammatory etiology, with lesions of the cerebral parenchyma later on. Also, electroencephalographic examinations in this case proved an evident perinatal lesion followed by degenerative changes.

2. S.J., boy, born 1956. The family history was not significant and the patient had no brothers or sisters. Delivery and development were normal. He suffered from all current children's diseases.

At the beginning of school attendance he started to blink his eyes abnormally, was restless, snorted and produced inarticulated sounds. He was very difficult to manage, several times having to interrupt school to be treated at the Department of Psychiatry. Since haloperidol treatment, he has been sociable. The neurological findings before six years of age spoke for minimal cerebral palsy, and today only a slight choreiform restlessness is present. Electroencephalogram shows accentuation of theta waves with hyperventilation, inclined to slight synchronization. Spinal fluid analysis showed the following: one lymphocyte and two polymorphonuclear leukocytes, protein 25 mg%, glucose 69 mg%, chlorides 418 mg%. Electrophoresis of fluid proteins showed albumin 64.6%, alpha/1, 5.6%, alpha/2, 6.2%, beta 12.8%, gamma 10.8% and A/G 1.63. Total serum protein was 7.36 gm%, with albumins 62.4%, alpha/1, 3.6%, alpha/2, 7.1%, beta 8.5%, gamma 18.4%, A/G 1.63. After any infection, the patient reveals a transitory clinical picture of generalized tics including coprolalia.

3. S.J., boy, born 1960. The father was strongly hyperactive in childhood and the mother is neurotic. He has no siblings. The mother suffered through the pregnancy badly, vomiting all the time, and delivery occurred three weeks early. Asphyxia appeared three hours after delivery, with improvement after application of oxygen. Severe infant jaundice was noticed. Development was retarded, as he started to speak only at the age of three years. He suffered from all common childhood infectious diseases. An average pupil at school, there has been worsening of school results recently.

The patient has squinted since birth, and in the second school grade he started to blink his eyes abnormally, after a month permanently hopping and twitching his shoulders. In 1969 he suffered a bad influenza, with fever lasting for nearly a month. In the period of convalescence, coprolalia appeared in addition to generalized tics. In February 1970, there was a recurrence of influenza with a significant worsening of tics. The neurological findings speak for cerebral palsy. The electroencephalogram shows imperfect maturation with increased paroxysmal readiness. The spinal fluid is Pandy negative, with 2 lymphocytes, protein 28 mg%, glucose 51 mg%, and chlorides 709 mg%. Spinal fluid proteins consisted of 57% albumin, 8.8% alpha/1, 8.8% alpha/2, 12.6% beta, and 12.8% gamma. Serum proteins totalled 5.8 gm%, with 61.2% albumin, 5% alpha/1, 10.5% alpha/2, 12.2% beta and 11.1% gamma.

There was an oscillating clinical course, worsening with infection, but the patient was sociable after the application of haloperidol.

Because of space limitations, only three case histories are presented. The other histories are available in summary.

In our series of 18 patients, there were 14 boys and four girls from the age of five up to 24 years, the average being 12 years. The period of observation was from 2-16 years. The family history was favorable in seven cases only. In the other cases there were tics in parents or brothers and sisters, stammering, enuresis or neurosis. Perinatal lesions were found in 14 cases due to premature or precipitated delivery, asphyxia, etc. All children were puking in the suckling period, were bad sucklings, slept little and were restless. They suffered from nearly all children's infectious diseases. The motor development was retarded in only four cases. Tics started at age three up to the age of 11 years, most frequently simultaneously with the start of school attendance around the age of seven. Most frequently observed in the beginning were abnormal blinking, grimaces, or licking one's lips. The localization of tics changed rather rapidly, some of them disappearing, some new appearing.

The clinical pictures are variegated and change before the observer's eyes. The children make an impression of marionettes that are quickly moved: they hop around all the time, the movements of extremities are very jerky, with brisk openings of mouth, flailing of knees, sharp turning of the trunk, the child never falling down. After several months respiration, tics, snuffling, snorting, coughing, or hissing appear. At this period, the children must interrupt school as they produce sounds very similar to animal voices, most often to the barking of a dog. At the beginning, the children speak in a normal way, their speech being plain except from time to time they produce an inarticulated sound. After several months, or days in some cases, they are afraid to speak as the inarticulated sounds multiply in their speech. The children are afraid to go to school, hold off from having friends, and are afraid even to go home as most parents at this period do not understand this is a disease and not a bad habit. The more the child is punished, the more quickly the tics spread, and the sooner coprolalia appears in addition. The children whose parents have understood the physician's advice and do not rebuke them for the tics, the course is much slighter and shorter, and in most cases the children need not interrupt their school attendance.

Most children, as said above, were strikingly restless since birth, but parents thought the reason for this was, as indicated, infectious diseases in 10 cases, injury in two cases, and tonsillectomy in two cases. In all children in our series, the tics worsened with any infection. The neurological findings were dependent on the period of examination. The younger the child, the sooner we could prove either the symptoms of minimal cerebral disease or of cerebral palsy. We found psychomotor maladroitness, choreiform restlessness, and differences both in the tonus and reflexes. An exception was the first case described, where the neurological findings worsened with growing age. In the other cases, pathological symptoms of the brain lesion were disappearing with growing age.

The electroencephalographic findings were clearly pathological in 15 cases. In most cases there was retarded electrical muturation, with stem dysfunction occurring in eight cases and increased paroxysmal readiness in four cases. The electroencephalographic picture, however, was improving, same as the clinical picture, with growing age, being temporarily worsened due to intercurrent infection. All the other auxiliary examinations — X-ray picture of the skull, fundus, urine, pediatric findings — were normal.

Electrophoresis of the spinal fluid could be performed in only five cases because in the other patients the protein content was so low that individual fractions could not be separated. Even the spinal fluid findings depend on the time of the tap. In children, after infections with an acute flare-up of the disease, spinal fluid examination spoke for inflammatory changes. In children with the chronic course or in remission we could find increased gamma globulins with a slight decrease of albumins and beta-globulins. The psychiatric and psychological evaluation will be presented by other authors. Until haloperidol appeared, the treatment had not been successful and only methophenazine (Frenolon) could make the patients substantially less restless. Since haloperidol has been used, all our patients have been sociable.

DISCUSSION

Itard (1825) and Sandras (1850) compared this disease to chorea. Bouteille, in **Traite de la Choree** (1818), complains that in this disease everything is rather strange: terms, symptoms, etiology and even the problematic therapy. There were really many terms. In 1880, Beard described "Jumpers of Maine"; in 1881, Friedreich speaks about "koordinierte Errinerungskrampfe"; in 1883, O'Brien published his article "Latah of Malaya"; and in 1884, Hammond presents his "myriachit of Siberia". Guinon, in 1886, speaks about "maladie des tics convulsifs"; in 1892, Marine speaks about "myospasia impulsiva" and in the same year Jolly described the "maladie des tics impulsifs". Chabbert, in 1893, is satisfied with the term "maladie des tics", but Brissaud in 1893 turns back to the original classification among the large group of choreas and suggests the term "choree polymorphe des degeneres." Bresler in 1896 separates a small subgroup under the term "mimischer Krampfneurose" and Koster in 1899 speaks about "motilitatsneurose".

A lot of authors were for a long period of time doubtful about the existence of this disease, some of them even thinking of simulation or pseudochorea with hysteric behaviour. It is interesting, nevertheless, that in as early as 1898 Wille explained the origin of this disease as being irritation of the nervous system with congenital or early acquired psycho- or neuropathic lesions of the brain.

Gilles de la Tourette, in 1885, characterized this disease of multiple tics, coprolalia, echolalia, and echokinesia. Both sexes were represented in the same amount of patients, sensitive individuals with hereditary histories prevailing.

More than 100 publications on this subject have appeared since his article was presented. There are not many discrepancies in the clinical evaluations. The start of the disease is generally indicated as being around 10 years of age. In more recent publications, the age in which the disease starts has been indicated as being even lower than 10 years. On one hand, Homburger (Boenheim, 1930) was still of the opinion that Gilles de la Tourette's disease does not appear in childhood; and on the other hand, MacDonald (1963) reported the start of the disease even in four-year-old patients, and Baker (1962) even in 3-5 year-old-children.

All authors agree in the observation that, at the very beginning of the disease, the tics were localized in the upper part of the body (68%), are increased with emotions and stress, decreased with intentness and in isolation, and absent in sleep. The course of the disease may be never foretold with certainty. It may slowly progress, completely stop, have paroxysmal exacerbations, or long-term remissions.

Tics in parents are very frequent.[198 222 45 153 149 145 243] The perinatal lesion is equally very frequent.[255 15 322 216 52] Retarded development was registered by Baker in 1962, enuresis by Ascher in 1948 and Morphew in 1969, and prevalence of ambidexters by Bockner in 1959.

The appearance of the disease following infectious diseases is pointed out by Brissaud (1896), Runger (1932), Ascher (1948), Heuscher (1950), Eisenberg (1959), Rapaport (1959), Magowska (1965), and Morphew (1969). Some authors think of the possibility of encephalitis.[142 14 372 52]

The neurological findings are, except for the multiple tics, mostly evaluated as normal, while some authors[162] always describe personality change. IQ varies from 87 (Ellison, 1964) up to 130 (Shapiro, 1968). They are mostly normal children.

The organic etiology of this disease has not been proven. Most authors point out psychogenic etiology. Guinon[207] speaks about psychic trauma, Bresler[62] about the irritation of the motor centers by psychic stimulus, and Koster[255] describes exhaustion of inhibitory and association centers evoked by chemical changes in the cells of degenerated individuals. Marchand[303] thinks of a congenital anomaly stopping the development of connections. According to this author, the molecular layer, in which the connections originate, is the area where, in certain conditions, the impulse initiating the performance of the tic originates. With maturation of the cells the tics disappear, but with infectious disease, interruption of connections, disturbance of balance, and recurrency of tics may occur.

DeWulf and Van Bogaert[136] exclude the organic etiology of Gilles de la Tourette's disease by section. Heuscher[221] is of the opinion that the patient sectioned by the above-mentioned authors did not at all suffer from this disease, as he was permanently psychically intact, the disease starting at the age of 18. There was no echolalia, no echokinesis and no hereditary history. Heuscher concludes that in this case the patient was impaired by tuberculosis and that there was imbalance in the activity of the basal ganglia. Kanner[241] speaks about the emotional trauma of degenerated persons. Ascher,[11] Hoefer and Kurland[264] point out the similarity with schizophrenia, Bockner[45] the obsedant neurosis, and Fenichel[164] the pregenital conversion. Hereditary histories are paid attention to by Koster,[255] Meige and Feindel,[316] Wilder,[485] and Bruch.[69]

The recent studies bridge the psychogenic and the organic etiologies. I. Magowska[293] speaks of the psychogenic superstructure in persons with organic lesions of the brain. Mazur[310] thinks of the hereditary idiopathic feebleness of corpus striati, rarely conditioned by an injury or infection, but with organic lesions always present. Brissaud,[64] Gerstmann and Schilder[192] and Mahler[297] speak about the constitutional inferiority of the subcortical structures. The possibility of disturbance of the basal ganglia and the stem already appears in the studies of Hammond,[213] Wilder,[485] Mahler[297] and Sulestrowska.[447]

On the basis of the electroencephalographic findings, Guggenheim[206] admits an affinity to epilepsy. Stevens and Blachly[441] do not exclude the metabolic dysfunction of the brain. Most modern authors admit that the etiology of Gilles de la Tourette's disease remains unclarified, and that there is very likely more than one cause.

The section findings have been, hitherto, very few. The normal findings of DeWulf and van Bogaert[136] has already been mentioned. Clauss and Balthasar[97] describe residual after meningitis, perivascular infiltrates and diffuse gliosis in their sectionally verified case. The maximum of the pathological findings was found in the basal ganglia and in the midbrain. Bing[39] also found thickening of meninges, but the brain of this patient was not histologically examined, and chronic meningitis could be present.

From the survey of the literature it appears that the patients with Gilles de la Tourette's disease are congenitally lesioned persons, mostly due to retarded maturation of the basal ganglia. The presupposition of organic etiology is confirmed by EEG findings as well. Both in EEG and in neurological examination the period when they were performed is very important. The younger the child, the more frequently we observe findings speaking for perinatal lesion. In the EEG there are clear signs of retarded maturation of the electrical activity, signs of stem dysfunction and sometimes even increased paroxysmal readiness. In elderly patients both the neurologic and EEG findings may be normal, which does not exclude an organic lesion of the basal ganglia, a fact which is well known. Normal EEG is described by Heuyer,[222] Michael,[322] Dunlap,[149] Milman,[324] Schneck,[410] Baker,[15] Bojanovski,[49] Challas,[84] Healy and Fischer,[216] Barsky,[20] Levy,[276] and Shapiro.[419]

Eisenberg[153] observed a patient with evidence for past encephalitis. The same was observed by Rapoport[383] and Koprowska-Milewska.[254] Increased paroxysmal readiness is described by Deshan,[132] Dolmierski,[143] Guggenheim,[206] and Kinnon.[312] Abnormal records without further specification are presented by Aimard,[5] Tobin and Reinhart,[452] Walsh,[473] Iio,[230] Kelman,[243] Magowska,[293] Faux,[161] Feild,[162] Stevens and Blachly,[441] Fernando,[168] Zgirski,[496] and Borak.[52]

MacDonald [289] describes a focus directly in the temporal lobe. In our series of patients, as already mentioned, the graph was clearly pathological in 15 cases. Normalization, *ie.,* maturation of electric activity, above all appeared with growing age, but signs of dysfunction of the stem or slight paroxysmal readiness survived. In three patients of our series, the electroencephalographic findings were normal, one of them being performed at the age of 12, the second at the age of 16, and the third at the age of 22 years. The result also depends on the total condition of the patient, the activity of the disease, the presence of infection, and the medications taken. This agrees with the findings of Kinnon. [312]

Examination of spinal fluid with normal findings is presented by Ascher,[11] Dunlap,[149] Baker,[15] Dolmierski,[142] Downing,[145] and Stevens.[441] In our series, the fluid findings were also mostly normal. Only in two patients, examined at the peak of their disease, was there a multiplication of cellules (36 up to 63). In the first patient, in whom there is no doubt about the organic character of the disease, proteins were also strikingly increased (146 mg%). On the other hand, the electrophoresis of proteins in the cerebrospinal fluid, if it could be performed at all due to the low percentage of proteins, was always more significant. In acute cases it spoke for inflammatory processes, while in chronic cases for a brain parenchyme lesion.

As far as the penumoencephalographic findings are concerned in the literature we found only a description of slight enlargement of the frontal apices [293] and of the asymmetric hydrocephalus. [52] We ourselves have performed this examination only in seven cases, three of which were normal. In three cases there was asymmetry of the ventricles and in one case there was atrophy of the cerebellum.

The therapy of this disease is, according to the literature, more difficult if compared with simple tics. Up to 1940 it did not, in fact, differ from the treatment of simple tics. Koster and Wille[255] tried diet and water therapy. Dunlap[149] suggests the free performance of the tic. Scopolamine and phenobarbital were not very successful,[136] and sleep treatment,[219] inhalation of CO_2,[322] and injections of novocaine[497] were also tried. A study by Feild[162] includes a survey of all ways of therapy until then: exercise, tranquilizers, sedatives, stimulants, anticonvulsants, antispasmodics, electric shocks, work therapy, psychotherapy, insulin shocks, lobotomy, and thalamotomy. With our series, we had good results with methophrenazine, but the best medication recognized today is haloperidol.[84 289 88 441 286 284 247 162 167 312 419]

Our results with haloperidol are also excellent. In agreement with Ford,[176] they are better the earlier the treatment is started, since at that age there are no personality changes.

If both our experiences and those indicated in the literature are summarized, we can conclude that:

1. Gilles de la Tourette's disease is conditioned by congenital inferiority of the basal ganglia, by the retarded maturation of the corpus striatum and thalamus and hence by the originating dysregulation of the excitation and inhibitory reactions.

2. In the history of these patients we find very often perinatal lesions and slight psychomotor retardation. The neurological findings in childhood prove a slight lesion of the brain. Also, EEG examination performed at this period proves retarded electric maturation.

3. The prognosis of this disease depends on many factors, above all on the rate of maturation of individual parts of the brain. In agreement with this rate are improvements in the electroencephalogram. After intercurrent diseases, infection, injuries, or psychic trauma, there is a substantial worsening, reflected in the EEG findings as well.

4. The organic origin of the disease is proved by both the EEG and psychologic examinations.[172] The examination of the spinal fluid is significant only at the very beginning of the disease (performed rather seldom, according to the literature), when it mostly speaks for an inflammatory etiology. Electrophoretic examination of the spinal fluid is very important, as it may prove both inflammatory etiology at the very beginning and a lesion of brain parenchyma in chronic cases.

5. The prognosis of the disease is not as poor as indicated by most authors. It may be due to the fact that today most patients have been treated earlier in childhood, and by a combination of modern psycho- and pharmacotherapy, the occurrence of irreversible changes is thus prevented. All of our patients, followed for many years, are sociable.

6. The dispute as to whether the etiology of this disease is psychogenic or organic does not seem to be substantial. Previously, epilepsy and chorea

were considered functional diseases, and it depends only on our diagnostic techniques, graphic and biochemical above all, when we succeed in revealing the basis of a certain disease. Also, with Gilles de la Tourette's disease, only complex, repeated examinations and a long-term following will help us to state the etiology and pathogenesis of this disease.

SUMMARY

The author summarizes her experiences with the long-term follow-up of 18 patients with the diagnosis of Gilles de la Tourette's disease, comparing them with data in the literature. She points out the frequency of the perinatal lesion of these patients, resulting both from the history of the patient, and the neurological as well as the encephalographic examination. The spinal fluid findings are pathological only at the very beginning of the disease, electrophoresis being much more significant. The prognosis depends on an early start of treatment and on secondary factors (trauma, infection, psychic lesion). Haloperidol is still a dominant medication in the treatment of this disease, with simultaneous correction of the family environment. It is supposed that the disease results from congenital inferiority of the basal ganglia, uneven maturation of individual nuclei and hence of originating dysregulation of excitation and inhibitory reactions.

Gilles de la Tourette's Syndrome. Volume 1: International Registry, p. 99-102, edited by F. Abuzzahab Sr. and F. Anderson. Mason Publishing Co., St. Paul ©1976.

A CASE REPORT
GILLES DE LA TOURETTE SYNDROME

Donald A. Galbraith, M.D., C.R.C.P.(C),
Director of Professional Education,
Children's Psychiatric Research Institute,
Clinical Assistant Professor of Psychiatry,
University of Western Ontario
London, Ontario, Canada

and

Timothy J. Turner,
Medical Student
University of Western Ontario
London, Ontario, Canada

Chapel, *et al.*, have noted that Gilles de la Tourette's disease is a syndrome of unknown etiology characterized by multiple vocal and motor tics tending to become worse under emotional stress.[88]

Almost every psychotropic drug and a variety of psychotherapeutic approaches have been utilized in the treatment of patients with this syndrome, with varying degrees of improvement noted. A recent review of literature in this regard has indicated that the greatest improvement has been achieved by the use of haloperidol.[430]

Fernando has noted that the rarity of Gilles de la Tourette syndrome is such that a review of published case reports is the only feasible method of surveying the broad aspects of the condition.[167]

The following case report is thus presented:

Identification

W.T. is a 32 year-old single Roman Catholic male who was first seen at age 13 by his family physician, because of frequent head shaking.

Social History

W. T. is the youngest of two boys of Yugoslavian parents. In early childhood he was exposed to many parental arguments and was often goaded into temper outbursts and then severely reprimanded. This resulted in a hostile, yet dependent relationship with his parents. His father saw his condition as a "bad habit" which could be "broken." He completed Grade 12 at the age of 18 and after attending college for one year he held a variety of jobs including clerk, computer operator and truck driver. He was engaged to a school teacher for several years but terminated the engagement shortly after his hospitalization in 1965.

History of Present Illness

After the onset of head shaking at age 13, W.T. was subsequently seen by several physicians before the diagnosis of Gilles de la Tourette's syndrome was made in 1962. During these years his symptom complex had expanded to include lip smacking, flexing of the left thumb, sniffling, barking, striking his temples with his fists, and in 1960 he began yelling short monosyllables such as "ma-ma" and "hey-hey." During the following two years his shouting increased markedly and coprolalia was reported in 1965 by an examining physician. However, evaluations of the patient since 1965 have not noted coprolalia. Between 1965 and 1968 W.T. was admitted to psychiatric hospitals on four occasions for treatment of 1 to 5 months duration.

Investigation

W.T.'s past medical history includes a tonsillectomy at age 7 for which he was completely unprepared and terrified and to which he attributes his initial development of "tics." Repeated physical evaluations have failed to show any significant abnormality and psyciatric assessments have failed to elicit any evidence of psychosis. On initial admission to the hospital in 1965 routine laboratory investigations were within normal limits. The EEG showed a low voltage record with no recognizable alpha rythm, beta activity present in all montages, and some scattered theta waves. There were no significant lateralizing or localizing features. Psychological testing at that time included the WAIS, Rosenzweig P-F study, M.M.P.I., Sacks Sentence Completion Test, the 16 Personality Factor Questionnaire, and T.A.T.W.T. obtained a full scale IQ of 78 and projective testing showed a passive dependent individual, who, "unable to express his hostilities openly, internalizes them or gives them expression through his symptoms."

Treatment

In February of 1961 W.T. was treated with thioridazine for a short period without success. In late 1964 outpatient psychotherapy combined with hypnosis was attempted. Failure of response resulted in a trial with haloperidol in November of 1964 but W.T.'s lack of cooperation in following the medication schedule and his increasing depression resulted in withdrawal of medication. In May, 1965 with his initial admission to hospital, W.T. was placed on several successive treatment regimes. Drug therapy included the use of chlorpromazine, propylthiouracil, niacin and combinations of chlordiazepoxide and isocarboxazid, chlorpromazine and amphetamine. His treatment also included two months of aversive conditioning and 9 interviews using initially sodium amobarbital and methamphetamine and later methamphetamine alone. The latter interviews revealed W.T.'s emotional immaturity and latent homosexuality. As well, they resulted in transient changes in personality and frequency of vocalizations. He was discharged November, 1965 on a treatment regime of chlorpromazine, amphetamine and ethopropazine with some improvement in his condition. W.T. was once again hospitalized in September of 1967 and his medication at that time had been changed to phenobarbital and procyclidine. He left the hospital after one month with his symptoms essentially unchanged from those of May, 1965, and returned January, 1968, at which time another intensive treatment program was instituted including lithium, haloperidol, and placebo, in conjunction with monitoring by a polygraph. However, symptomatology remained unchanged, and W.T. was discharged after two months with the advice that he would have to "live with his symptoms."

Current Status

Interview in July of 1970 with W.T. revealed basically unchanged patterns of muscular tics, blowing and sniffing, interspersed with yells and barks. He is presently on no medication and while living with his parents he has been able to work as a truck driver.

CONCLUSION

This case substantiates the generalizations made by Chapel regarding the absence of evidence of organicity and the presence of family pathology.[167]

Despite extensive psychiatric treatment, including the use of haloperidol, this patient has shown no lasting improvement; however, at present he is able to function outside of hospital.[86]

Gilles de la Tourette's Syndrome. Volume 1: International Registry, p. 103-115, edited by F. Abuzzahab Sr. and F. Anderson. Mason Publishing Co., St. Paul ©1976.

TOURETTE'S DISEASE AS A CLINICAL MODEL FOR THERAPEUTIC RESEARCH: LONGITUDINAL CASE STUDY # 1

Walter Knopp, M.D.,
Professor

and

Marilyn Strayer, M.D.,
Clinical Instructor
The Ohio State University, College of Medicine,
Department of Psychiatry,
Columbus, Ohio 43210 U.S.A.

Recently, the tragedy of Tourette's disease (T.D.) has been well described by Shapiro, *et al.*[418] In its dimensions it can be compared only to the tragedy of **physical** death due to cancer and of **social** death due to some forms of the schizophrenias. Fortunately, in T.D., many patients, although not all of them, can be symptomatically improved by the butyrophenone haloperidol.

This is the first in a series of graphically documented clinical observations and quantitative evaluations attempting to study the effects of drugs and related and unrelated factors upon the therapeutic response or lack of it of the individual patient. Similar to the schizophrenias, intra- and interpersonal factors are of utmost importance in T.D. However, the target symptom of the latter can be directly observed and more reliably measured under double blind conditions. By employing a multi-disciplinary approach we hope to have made one little step toward a more detailed understanding of the complex interplay between endogenous and exogenous forces. Eventually a more rational therapeutic approach to T.D. and, perhaps, to the much more frequent group of schizophrenias may evolve.

SUBJECT

The patient was born in 1949 after a normal pregnancy by an uneventful although induced forceps delivery. He began teething and sitting up at about 6 months, walking at 10 months, and talking at 18 months of age. No feeding difficulties were reported.

At 9 months the patient had mumps, at 2 years whooping cough and all through his early childhood he had frequent sore throats which prompted a tonsillectomy at 4. He had chicken pox the same year. At 5 he had pneumonia and measles when he was 8. Nocturnal enuresis was last reported at 15. On admission to our hospital there was no significant family history except for a paternal cousin who was a patient in a child guidance setting.

At 2½ the patient's parents began noting strange repetitive movements such as picking at his right shoulder or at his shirt. Different doctors advised the parents not to worry and to wait until the patient outgrew those habits.

By 4 years of age the patient started shaking his head from side to side and also was exhibiting some abnormal hand movements. These movements gradually progressed in severity and extent involving the patient's entire body. When the patient was 7 years old the family moved to another city of about the same size (30,000), about 130 miles west of his home town.

During his early school years the patient attended regular classes most of the time. Most of his difficulties started in the 7th grade when he was about 12 years old. He began having difficulties sitting still in class and his classmates began to ridicule him. This became more complicated when his muttered guttural noises developed into a frank coprolalia when he was upset. Among his numerous actions was a characteristic tic of sticking out his tongue, followed or associated with spitting. The patient began losing his temper and kept getting into fights. When he was almost 13 (1962), he underwent extensive neurological and child psychiatric examinations at an internationally noted hospital. By that time, however, five or six EEG's were reportedly found within normal limits except for one of them. The patient has been treated by various sedatives, tranquilizers and diphenylhydantoin to no avail. A few quotes may illustrate the patient's behavior at that time: "The tics are indeed multiple and cannot be controlled. They significantly include throat tics with occasional ejaculation of sounds such as "Cha-cha-cha-cha". . . (the patient) is a pleasant, cooperative youngster, understandingly puzzled about himself as he says: there are so many crooks and criminals and they don't have anything like this, but it had to happen to me. . . About the only thing to do is to have him continue in school where the teachers are aware of his problem and are reasonably considerate. Some form of medication should be given since he does hope for some beneficial effect.

The director of the epilepsy clinic to whom the patient was originally referred for consultation wrote as follows: "This patient presents a very difficult diagnostic problem and I must admit that I cannot come to a decision as to a specific diagnosis at this time. However, I do believe that the symptomatology simulates the syndrome of Gilles de la Tourette more than any other disorder I can think of . . .I am at a loss to recommend therapy in this case at this time." The consultant did not believe that psychiatric therapy would be of any avail, and that the parents and the patient would have to learn how to live with this disorder. "The mother was very much in favor of my trying some type of medication; therefore, I started the patient on one of our new experimental anticonvulsants. . . ."

Subsequently, the patient was taken out of school and tutored privately. In 1963 he spent six months in a private boarding hospital school designed for hyperkinetic mentally retarded children. However, the patient at that time showed a verbal IQ of 110 and performance IQ of 107 and a full scale IQ of 109. The authorities felt that although the patient benefitted from the kindly inpatient atmosphere, he needed a special school where the environment was conducive to active psychiatric treatment. They recognized that it would be exceedingly difficult for the patient to attend regular public schools under the circumstances. In their opinion the patient's parents seemed to be "good parents" but "just unable to grasp the full significance of their child's illness."

Shortly after discharge from the boarding hospital-school the patient had another psychological evaluation. When he was almost 14 years of age: "To date no constructive treatment has been arranged for (the patient) in spite of extensive diagnostic studies." The patient was now on home tutoring but not under treatment. He has trouble going to sleep. He first inspects the bed, then after he is in he beats himself. He is enuretic once per week. Occasionally he complains of dizziness. He has many tics including protruding his tongue. He is practically 9th grade but is on home tutoring.

Mother describes herself as flying off the handle . . . . (and) backward with people. Father feels that his wife is the best in the world. He makes friends easily. He has a bad temper. He worries about his business, the bills and the patient. Because he had so little in his childhood, he showers things on both of his sons. The patient's brother, aged 17, does average in school, has many friends and loves sports. He is kind to the patient but resists including him in his games.''

In summary, the psychological report strongly recommended that the patient be admitted to a state children's psychiatric hospital. Subsequently, the patient was admitted to such a (dynamically oriented) hospital where he stayed for about 18 months. He was treated by individual psychotherapy and milieu treatment. "An attempt was made to work out his hostility toward his parents. He began using vulgar words in a repetitive fashion which further troubled his parents and often caused open conflict. . . . Our diagnosis was obsessive-compulsive neurosis.'' The parents were described as overprotective and infantilizing and the father as an obsequious person, manipulative and preoccupied with his own background of deprivation and rejection. The patient was discharged with the understanding that he would continue seeing his psychotherapist who joined a local state hospital near the patient's home town. At that time haloperidol became available on an experimental basis. However, the patient's therapist was not allowed to use experimental drugs and, therefore, referred the patient to us.

METHODS AND RESULTS

The patient was admitted to the psychiatric wing of the Ohio State University Hospitals on October 25, 1965, and he remained hospitalized until May 28, 1966. After a non-blind observation period of three weeks a double blind cross-over longitudinal study was begun with one week of placebo (Figure 1). (Some aspects of our methodology have been described previously).[85 250] Thereafter, the patient was treated by gradually increasing doses of haloperidol up to 11 mgs per day. In the 17th week the placebo was abruptly substituted for the active drug, on March 15, 1965. The plan was to withdraw the drug for a total of three weeks; however, the response of the patient, as well as of his treatment team was so dramatic that haloperidol was resumed (again on double blind basis) after only one week. Haloperidol was again increased up to a total of 10 mgs daily and continued until May 16 at the beginning of the 26th week when placebo was again substituted for haloperidol. Again the patient became depressed assuming that haloperidol lost its effect. The ward personnel became panicky and I had no choice but either telling the truth and thus break the code, restarting haloperidol or **dampen** the emotional impact by a minor tranquilizer on May 21, 1965 in the form of diazepam, 5 mgs three times daily which the patient has received ever since.

In addition to haloperidol, which was given double blindly, the patient received other medications as indicated and as ordered by his treating

FIGURE 1

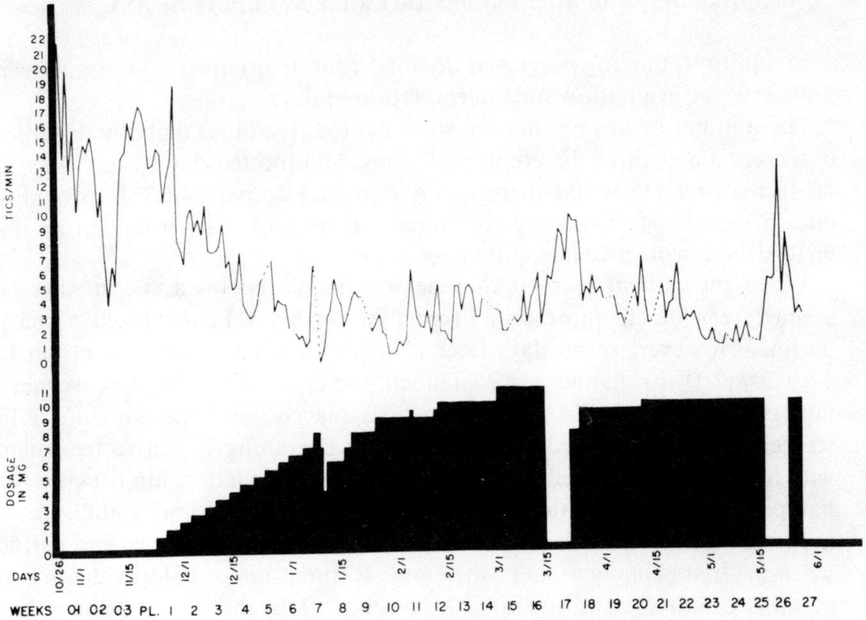

Relationship between haloperidol intake and target symptom frequency.

The abscissa represents the actual dates as well as the weeks of study. 0.1, 0.2, and 0.3 denote weeks of non-blind observation; PL, 17 and 26, the placebo weeks. The rest of the numbers indicate the haloperidol weeks of the double blind part of the study. All designations are placed in the middle of each week.

The lower ordinate indicates haloperidol dosage in milligrams per day and the upper ordinate the average tic frequency per minute. The dashed lines indicate days on which no rating took place.

physician, usually consisting of chloral hydrate at bedtime, phenobarbital, 30 mg as needed from 1 to 4 times daily, nose drops or oral decongestants, antibiotics, and from May 5 on trihexyphenidyl, 1 mg b.i.d., without visible effects on the measured parameters. In addition to routine laboratory tests, as they were required with the use of an experimental drug, the patient's 24 hour urine was collected twice weekly beginning with the placebo week for 12 weeks. The 24 hour urine samples were collected to determine the 24 hour excretion rate of norepinephrine (NE), dopamine (DA) and their major acid metabolites vanillylmandelic acid (VMA) and homovanilic acid (HVA) respectively.[319] For this reason the patient received a vanilla- and xanthine-free diet from November 8, 1965 for a total of 12 weeks. The orders were written and the patient was told on November 5. However, the diet was actually started on November 8.

To study the inter-relationships between behavioral observations, neurophysiological measurement, biochemical measures and drug intake the following methods were used:

1. Target symptom changes in terms of a tic frequency (T.F.) per minute.
2. Planimetric determination of handwriting area (PDHA).

3. Electronic pupillography (EPG).
4. Gorham-Overall Brief Psychiatric Rating Scale (GO-BPRS).

In addition, nursing notes and doctors' routine progress notes have been utilized in the evaluation and interpretation of data.

The number of tics per minute was counted five times daily by different observers under three different conditions, and plotted day by day (Figure 1). In the first 1½ weeks there was a moderate decrease of T.F. probably due to the change from the emotionally laden home environment to the neutral and protective hospital milieu.

When the patient learned that he will be placed on a special diet he seemed very much impressed. From here on his T.F. displayed a sharp decline. However, seven days later it began to climb again. He began to verbalize: "If the diet helps me so much, the first pill is going to cure me." However, the first pill happened to be a placebo and the patient's T.F. seemed slightly increased again. From the beginning of active treatment with haloperidol there seems to be an almost 1 to 1 relationship between the haloperidol dosage and tic frequency. As the dosage becomes stabilized the negative trend levels off and it is sharply interrupted by the placebo period when the trend changes to a positive one. Resumption of haloperidol brings about a negative trend again with leveling off in the weeks prior to the second placebo period. The latter changes the trend again abruptly into a positive one while resumption of haloperidol does again the opposite.

In the monitoring of the extrapyramidal motor activity, we used our previously described PDHA. The patient was instructed under standard conditions to copy a four line verse three times within four minutes. We used the nursery rhyme — "Jack and Jill went up the hill, etc . . . " This procedure was repeated each day, the area occupied by each verse was measured, the median selected, and plotted day by day.

Figure #2 displays the trends of the PDHA, *i.e.*, handwriting size. They are very similar to those displayed by the T.F., except on two occasions, which were associated with periods of intense emotional upheavals. The marked increases in the 4th and 5th haloperidol weeks coincided with the emotionally laden Christmas time and the fact that the patient was very disappointed about the possibility of having to discontinue haloperidol because of a pathological liver function test. As soon as he learned that the latter was a laboratory error, his handwriting size returned to the expected lower level, on December 28th and 29th, 1965. The less marked increases in the 6th and 7th week coincided with the year-end activities which in turn were followed by an irritation of the patient's left eye and a beginning akathisia, because of which the haloperidol dosage had to be decreased transiently. From about the 15th of January the handwriting size remained well below the level of his pre-drug handwriting size. However, the day-to-day oscillations became more pronounced, as did the patient's emotional status, which was subject to quite intensive mood swings from day to day and week to week. Getting used to a life without tics posed many problems which

FIGURE 2

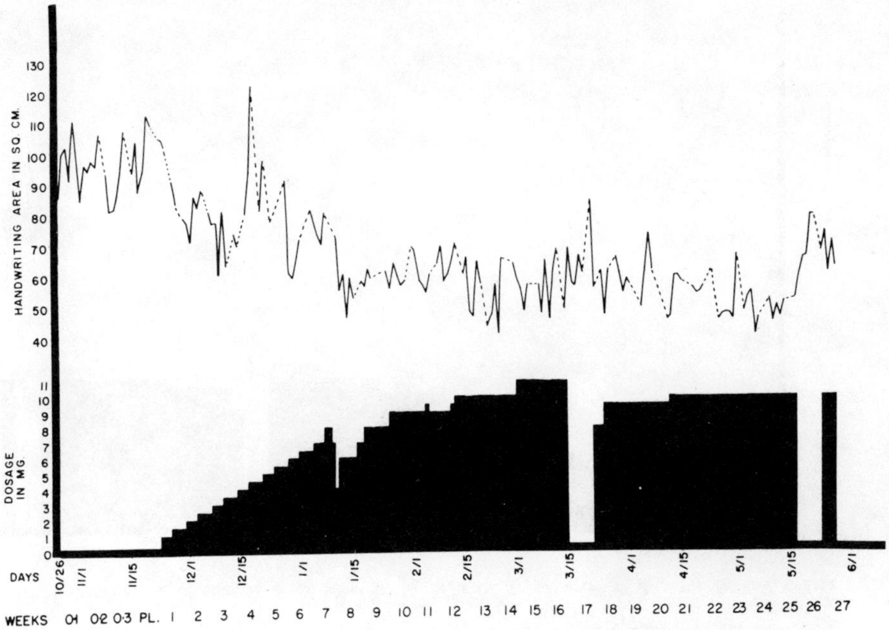

Relationship between haloperidol intake and handwriting size (planimetric determination of handwriting area).

The abscissa represents the actual dates as well as the weeks of study. 0.1, 0.2, and 0.3 denote weeks of non-blind observation; PL, 17 and 26, the placebo weeks. The rest of the numbers indicate the haloperidol weeks of the double blind part of the study. All designations are placed in the middle of each week.

The lower ordinate indicates haloperidol dosage in milligrams per day and the upper ordinate the average handwriting area in square centimeters. The dashed lines indicate days on which no testing took place.

needed psychological treatment, by group and individual psychotherapy, as well as milieu therapy. Because of the quite extensive day-to-day oscillations, the response to the first placebo week (the 17th week) is not very dramatic. Even after resumption of haloperidol the intense oscillation remained until about two weeks before the 2nd placebo week, at which time the handwriting size showed quite a dramatic change of trend upward followed by a downward trend upon the resumption of haloperidol as expected.

The GO-BPRS (Figure 3) was used single blindly at irregular intervals by one of us (W.K.). Similar to the T.F. and PDHA, the GO-BPRS scores declined sharply in the beginning of the haloperidol period. Thereafter there was no resemblance to T.F. except in the 26th week and to PDHA in the 4th, 5th and 26th week of haloperidol treatment.

In EPG, under standard conditions and after standard dark adaptation, standard light stimuli were presented in the form of a .1 second light stimulus, followed by a 4.9 second darkness. Five values were averaged and

FIGURE 3

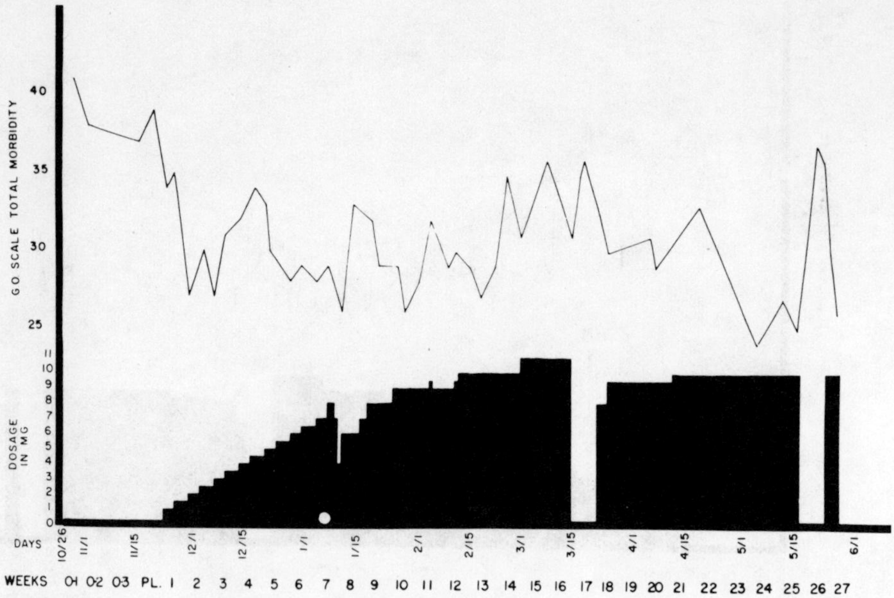

Relationship between haloperidol intake and the Gorham-Overall Brief Psychiatric Rating Scale (total morbidity).

The abscissa represents the actual dates as well as the weeks of study. 0.1, 0.2, and 0.3 denote weeks of non-blind observations; PL, 17 and 26, the placebo weeks. The rest of the numbers indicate the haloperidol weeks of the double blind part of the study. All designations are placed in the middle of each week.

The lower ordinate indicates haloperidol dosage in milligrams per day and the upper ordinate the total morbidity scores of the GO Scale.

the results plotted daily. Figure 4 displays the pupillary findings. The upper curve shows the dark adapted diameter of the pupil. Although quite extensive fluctuations have taken place which remind one of the fluctuations seen in the PDHA, no visible trend perturbation coincides with the beginning of haloperidol treatment or dosage changes. The lower curve shows the extent of pupillary contraction (EC). During the observation and placebo periods the pupil's EC fluctuated about an average of approximately .3 mm. As soon as haloperidol medication was started, the EC increased almost three-fold. For the following seven weeks the EC fluctuated about an average of approximately .6 mm and then gradually the trend decreased to about an average of .5 mm, except for the extensive perturbation of trend at the time of a dose adjustment in the 20th week.

All through his stay in our hospital attempts have been made to have the patient participate regularly at a nearby private school, which the patient successfully avoided and eventually gave up entirely. However, his general social adjustment improved markedly by end of April, 1966. His emotional upheavals and oscillations in T.F. and PDHA became less intense and he himself felt more relaxed, self-confident and ready to leave our hospital and

FIGURE 4

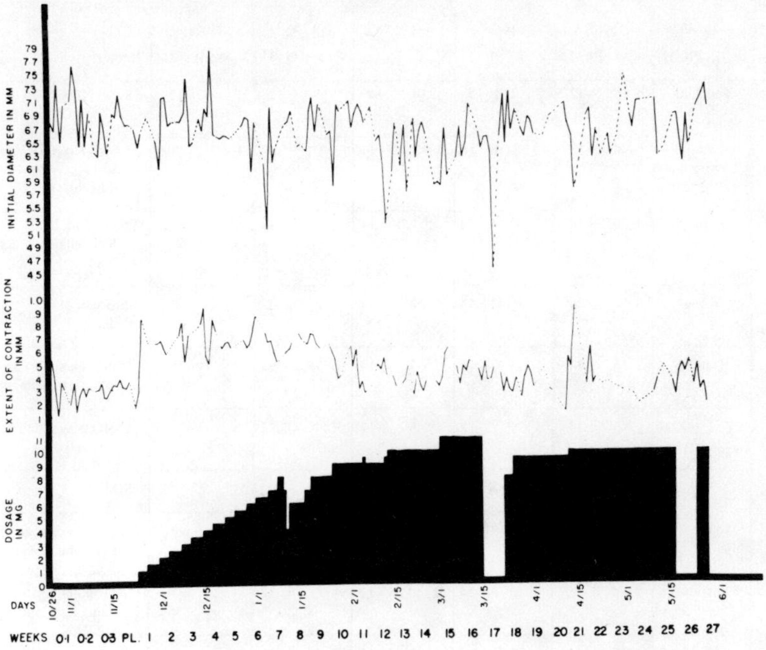

Relationship between haloperidol intake and the electronic pupillography.

The abscissa represents the actual dates as well as the weeks of study. 0.1, 0.2, and 0.3 denote weeks of non-blind observations; PL, 17 and 26, the placebo weeks. The rest of the numbers indicate the haloperidol weeks of the double blind part of the study. All designations are placed in the middle of each week.

The lower ordinate indicates haloperidol dosage in milligrams per day, the middle ordinate the extent of pupillary contraction in millimeters (*i.e.*, the largest diameter of the resting dark-adapted pupil). The dashed lines indicate days on which no tests were performed.

begin a summer job before returning to school in the fall of 1966. This appeared to be the last chance to replicate the findings generated by the first placebo substitution. As expected, the patient and the staff reacted dramatically to their assumption that haloperidol lost its therapeutic effect. Resumption of haloperidol 10 mg daily promptly returned the situation to the pre-placebo level of adjustment and the patient was indeed discharged after four more days.

FIVE YEAR FOLLOW-UP

Table 1 summarizes the most important aspects of treatment to date (March, 1971). After discharge, the patient's family situation has stabilized to a degree unknown to them in the past 14 years. The patient continued to be followed on out-patient basis. At first he was tutored at home and towards the end of 1967 he returned to the public school where he graduated one year behind his class in June, 1968. Brief outpatient visits usually

TABLE 1

	1966				1967				1968				1969				1970				1971				
	V	T	Ph	H	V	T	Ph	H	V	T	Ph	H	V	T	Ph	H	V	T	Ph	H	V	T	Ph	H	Remarks
JAN	Psychiat				4	16		12.5	2	3	2	14	1	10		14				12				12	*Surg. Hosp. x 10 days H 7 mg x 3 days
FEB	Hospital				5	6		13	1	2	6	14	1	3		14				12	1	3		12	**Psych.Hosp. x16 days MMPI Congention
MAR	10-25-65				4	9		14	1	0		14				14				12				12	***prostate Rohrschach TAT
APR	through				3	4	1	14		*	1	14	1	8	+	14	1	1		12					y quit school — orderly
MAY	5-28-66				2	6		14	1	3		14	1	3		14	1	1		12					yy Surg. Hosp. x4 days Endo. Hosp. x8 days
JUN	2	1		10				14	1	6		14	1	8		14				12					yyy Starts as Inhal. therapist
JUL	2	3		11	1	9		14			4	14	1	3	**	10-14	1	8		12					z MMPI
AUG	3	4		11	2	5		16	1	4		14	4	5	***	10-12				12					zz Upset by change of H. schedule
SEPT	3	4		11	1	4	1	16	1	12		14	2	1	y	12	yyy		1	12					zzz Troubles with fiancee's family
OCT	3	5		12	1	5		16	1	5		14	1	3		12	1	5	z	12					+ Surg. Hosp. x6 days
NOV	4	9		12	2	5	3	14	2	9		14		yy	3	12	zz		1	12					
DEC	4	2		12	2	3		14	1	10		14				12				12					

Legend: V = # of Visits Ph = # of phone calls
T = Tics per minute H = Haloperidol im mg/day

Five year follow up: frequency of office visits and phone calls per month, frequency of tics per minute (during most tense moments of the office visits) and daily dosage of haloperidol.

consisted of drug adjustments and at times, help with emotional readjustment to life at school, jobs, and leisure, as well as conferences with his teachers and parents. Any attempt to "probe deeper" was met with increased tension. Supportive therapy and crisis intervention were the most successful techniques employed. The dosage of haloperidol had to be increased gradually up to 14 mg daily, supplemented by diazepam 5 mg daily, to "take the edge off" the patient's emotional and social readjustments. On one occasion his cephalin flocculation reaction was 3+ with a prompt decrease to trace the next month. Otherwise there have been no alarming pathological laboratory findings. Only for brief periods while in his senior year of high school his dosage had to be increased to 16 mgs daily. His vital signs have been within normal limits, except for brief periods of "colds" at which times his pulse was above average and blood pressure below. Shortly before his graduation elective surgery (rhinoplasty) was performed for which the haloperidol dosage was decreased transiently to 7 mgs daily. The elective surgery was tolerated without untoward effect.

After graduation the patient had to go through another series of difficult readjustments. Although he intended at one time to go to college he finally decided to take a vocational school like his father and brother, both of whom were barbers at that time. However, there were some difficulties in securing a placement for the patient. He worked as a grave digger at one time, later secured a job in a filling station. Socially and occupationally he had difficulties with his quick temper as described above.

The year 1969 was an especially difficult year for the patient. In April, one year after his first elective surgery, he entered the hospital to have "bone chips" removed from his knee joint. Again the same haloperidol dose adjustment was transiently made as one year earlier, and the surgery was tolerated without untoward effect.

On July 1, 1969, he was readmitted to our hospital because of bouts of being tense, anxious and angry, with pallor, sweating and tachycardia. These spells lasted about three minutes. The patient also complained of blurred vision, being worse at night, with objects appearing large and fuzzy. The spells occurred at any time and were not precipitated by anything known to the patient.

The physical examination and laboratory data, including EEG with thorough ophthalmological examination with ERG, were found to be normal. An MMPI profile appeared to be within normal limits but with some inconsistencies within his pattern. In the hospital he had only one spell immediately upon admission, when he became very nervous and agitated, his face flushed, with normal pulse and blood pressure. The patient was able to recognize the probability of an emotional upset "for a good reason." When the threat dissipated he improved immediately and was anxious to return home.

After another month with genito-urinary irritation, the patient decided to give up the idea of entering a vocational school and decided to take a job as an orderly in his home town. In November, 1969, he was again admitted for a "vague pain in the costovertebral area." After reassurance that all his physical complaints are not related to a rather high haloperidol dosage, he began to display a gradual upward trend socially and vocationally. Although the average T.F. on occasions was as high as before haloperidol, their range never reached the pre-haloperidol values (5-70 per minute), nor did their intensity. Now, his T.F. decreased to a minimum and those few tics still remaining were hardly noticeable. In September, 1970, he advanced to the position of an inhalation therapist at a large metropolitan hospital. Another short-lasting but intense upheaval followed, precipitated by rejecting attitudes on the part of his future in-laws. He was able to resolve constructively the issues involved, became engaged and plans to get married in September, 1971.

DISCUSSION

Very interesting relationships are revealed when the values and the trends of the 24-hour excretion rates of catecholamines and their metabolites is compared with TF, PDHA and EPG.[319] DA excretion was above normal prior to and on small doses of haloperidol. Prolonged haloperidol treatment (up to the 10th week) was associated with a decrease in DA excretion toward normal levels, corresponding to the decrease in TF and PDHA. The HVA and NE trends appear to be reciprocal to those of EPG, EC, while VMA trends are similar to those of the dark-adapted pupil. These findings may have far reaching implications of theoretical significance.[319 381 430 248 249] Also, a very interesting observation was made at the time of the second placebo substitution in the 26th week. As indicated in Figure 5, the decrease in TF and PDHA began on 5-21-66, *i.e.*, before

FIGURE 5

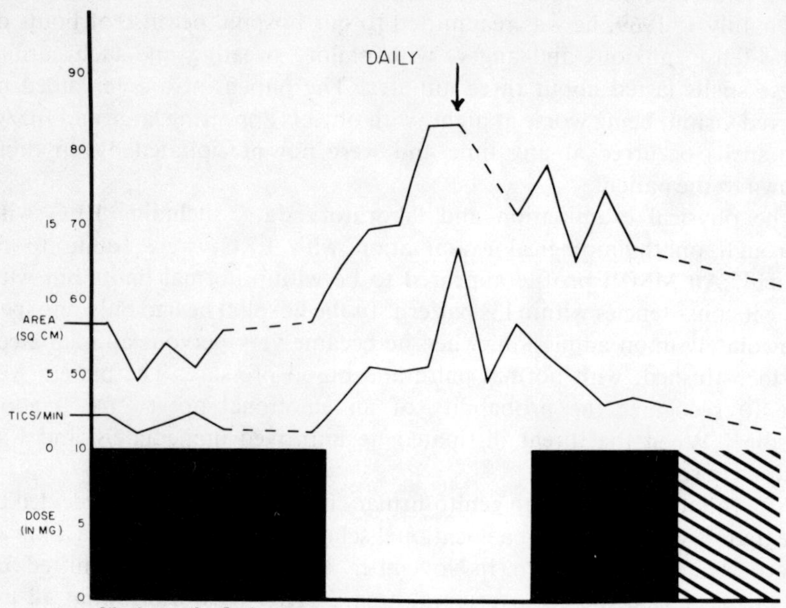

Enlarged version of the second placebo period, displaying the relationship between haloperidol intake, tic frequency and handwriting area. The abscissa represents the actual dates and the lower ordinate the haloperidol dosage in milligrams per day. The two upper ordinates display tic frequency per minute and handwriting area in square centimeters. Beginning May 21 diazepam (arrow), 5 mg three times daily was added to the haloperidol schedule.

haloperidol was resumed and coincidental with the beginning of diazepam treatment. As mentioned above, the patient was extremely upset, to have his tics returned in all violence so close to his discharge. To counteract his emotional reaction we added diazepam. A distinct difference in the action of diazepam as compared to haloperidol was noticed.

While taking diazepam, the patient was able to willfully suppress his tics for a limited period of time — that is, the time of testing, when he felt observed and rated. Once the motivation to suppress them was gone, the tics returned in all violence. While on haloperidol, the patient had no need to suppress the tics, for none were present.

In conclusion, it seems that individual patient-oriented and objective monitoring of drug treatment in neuropsychiatry is possible. However, neither descriptions and movies nor graphs can give full account of the emotional struggle within the patient, and of the psycho-social measures applied by the treatment team. Both were important parts of the treatment once the drug had removed the tic as a major problem in his relationship with people. In two subsequent case studies we shall demonstrate the reliability of this procedure and introduce some perspectives regarding the use of similar procedures in monitoring the drug effects in the treatment of a vastly more frequent debilitating disease — schizophrenia.

ACKNOWLEDGMENT

This study has been supported by the NIH General Research Development Grant administered by the Ohio State University College of Medicine and the Psychiatric Research Foundation of Columbus. Haloperidol was generously supplied by McNeil Laboratories, Inc.

The authors wish to express their appreciation to the many professional, technical and administrative staff members without whose contribution this complex study could not have been accomplished.

Gilles de la Tourette's Syndrome. Volume 1: International Registry, p. 117-122, edited by F. Abuzzahab Sr. and F. Anderson. Mason Publishing Co., St. Paul ©1976.

GILLES DE LA TOURETTE'S SYNDROME

Elzbieta Koprowska-Milewska, M.D.
Specialist in General and Child Psychiatry
Katowice, ul.
Bankowa 27/79, Poland

Although the etiology of Gilles de la Tourette's syndrome is still in question, for an increasing majority of authors it seems to be a specific complex of symptoms that are due to injuries of determinate structures of the subcortex.

Charcot[90 93] treated tics primarily like psychogenic disturbances while Trousseau,[458] who described the various forms of the tics, referred to their organic background and was the first to describe echolalia and coprolalia accompanying the tics. A student of Charcot, Gilles de la Tourette,[198] was the first to select from the wide variety of dyskinesias, a complex consisting of compulsive movements, appearing mainly among the facial, lingual and acromial muscles, and various symptoms of repetition, including echolalia, echopraxia and arithmomania. Also seen were vocal symptoms of a compulsive nature, like inspirations, expirations, hissing, and utterances of nonarticulated sounds or obscene words, suggesting their psychogenic origin. The observation of tics in animals,[351 352] showing the similar symptoms of sudden contracting around the face, neck and shoulders together, coupled with the observations of compulsive movements accompanied by pallilalia in the course of the hyperkinetic form of epidemic encephalitis speaks for the organic background of the tic syndrome. The relationship of the postencephalitic conditions appears strong in view of the fact that the behavioral disturbances in Gilles de la Tourette's syndrome and Economo's encephalitis proved to be almost identical with prevalence in both conditions of intense impulsivity, retarded affect, high irritability and the psychosomatic proneness to fatigue.

Microscopic evidence of the organic origin of Tourette tics was presented in the anatomopathological papers of Clauss and Balthasar.[97 18] The histological changes were of two kinds. The first changes noted were hypoplasia of the cells in the corpus striatum with an increase in the number of small cells to large cells in the striatum, similar to the cellular picture in the infant. The number and density of small striatal cells in a 42-year-old patient corresponded approximately to the striatum in a one-year-old infant. It is the opinion of Balthasar that the insufficient maturity of the striatum is responsible for reduced coordination of cortical activity by the basal ganglia.

The second group of anatomopathological changes was typical of those left after meningoencephalitis with glial prolifereration in the lateral paracentral thalmus and cell destruction, most marked in the cortex.

Tics may arise after scarlet fever, diptheria and angina, but most commonly after rheumatic disease (chorea minor).[444 445 112] The Soviet authors[259] agree that, besides chorea minor, rheumatic disease can produce changes in the central nervous system which cause other hyperkinetic symptoms, particularly often tics. Diagnosis can be difficult in these forms, particularly when changes of behavior, suggesting neurosis, are observed. In 33 patients, aged from 5-15 years, with various forms of rheumatic encephalitis were seen at the Institute of Neurology in Moscow, 13 were found to be suffering from hyperkinetic symptoms.[259] Twelve of these were found to have had protracted angina or tonsillitis. The tics involved the muscles of the face, palate, neck and shoulders. It is of note that the same muscles were involved as in Tourette's syndrome, and that the tics' intensity varied with activity and stress, disappearing during sleep. Symptoms included oculogyration, grimacing, inarticulations and neck and arm tics.

These movements could be distinguished from the typical uncoordinated choreatic movements in various parts of the body by absent or only slightly reduced muscle tonus, involvement of the same muscles or muscle groups, and rapid, brusque nature. According to the Soviet authors, the anatomic injury in the above quoted cases was mainly in the basal ganglia, but also in the secondary cortex, and developed as a diffuse vascular process.

The development and course of the hyperkinetic forms of rheumatic encephalitis may vary. With some patients the hyperkinesis develops acutely after angina and flu, sometimes along the joint components, and the symptoms remain for several months, regressing slowly. In other cases, the malady assumes a protracted course from the very beginning, with periodic arthralgia, endocarditis and exacerbation of the hyperkinesis in the interim. Such a protracted, continuous character was observed by Kucemilowa[259] with patients showing rheumatic encephalitis in the tic form.

In the Polish literature Bilikiewicz[35] considers that the majority of tics are due to psychogenic reasons, that their presence is the consequence of a psychic injury and that they are responsive to psychotherapy. The frequent tics, however, like movement neurosis, may be responsible for obscuring the organic background. Sulestrowski and Wdowiak[448] refer to the organic injury as being responsible for the tics and the obsessional neurosis.

In the cases that were subject to further investigation in Poland, the authors were of the opinion that Gilles de la Tourette's syndrome is of organic nature. In the report from the Gdansk Infirmary,[142] febrile episodes including a convulsive episode, were observed in one patient. These episodes were exacerbated by a smallpox vaccination. Also, the symptoms of a psychological complex were observed in the boy, and distinct electroencephalographic changes were localized in the temple. In another case, the evidence for organic background was not confirmed by the history, but the psychological complex (light euphoria, irritability and affective imbalance) was seen, the intelligence was low, and electroencephalographic pathology was found at the temples. In both cases the condition of the patients improved with chlorpromazine, which acts mainly in the brain stem and subcortical nuclei. The tics returned when the drug was discontinued.

In 1959, a case of Gilles de la Tourette's syndrome was described,[378] the patient being a nine-year-old boy who had contracted rheumatic disease with chorea and endocarditis. The electroencephalogram showed generalized changes, and an asymmetric deep tendon reflex pattern was found in the neurological examination. Intelligence was normal. Treatment included chlorpromazine, phenobarbital and narcoanalysis. The involuntary movements disappeared after five months, but the compulsive vocalizations continued.

In two cases of the syndrome at the Psychiatric Hospital in Lubliniec reported in 1966,[254] we also suggested an organic etiology. In the first patient, S.G., the parents described a severe case of hematopoietic flu followed by tics. While hospitalized, disturbances in behavior consisting of intense impulsivity and irritability were seen, but no evidence of motor or vocal tics was observable. The electroencephalogram was pathologic. Since his discharge his progress in school was very slow, and tics and vocal symptoms appeared and were treated with some improvement. From 1964-1971, the patient was hospitalized eleven times for Tourette's syndrome, and his symptomatology variously included throwing things around, aggressive behavior, disturbances of sleep, and an offensive approach to girls in public places (even his own sister).

The second case we reported was that of a girl, K.J., who, after the acute attack of rheumatic fever ceased, developed motor tics with coprolalia and an abnormal encephalogram. Treatment with chlorpromazine and salicylates resulted in periodic relief, although the tics returned with rheumatic pain or angina. From the outpatient as well as inpatient pediatric population with hyperkinesis we have learned that the pattern of Gilles de la Tourette's syndrome is extremely variable, and this has persuaded us to publish the following report.

CASE REPORTS

In 1970 there were two cases of Gilles de la Tourette's syndrome observed in the Department of Developmental Psychiatry in Lubliniec. The first patient, P.M., born on the 7th of July, 1958 was referred from the child psychiatry outpatient department in Katowice with the following history:

During the pregnancy the mother took quinine and alcohol with the intention of inducing an abortion. She was beaten several times while quarrelling with her husband. The boy was born without complications. He fell twice from the divan to the floor at two and four months of age, though in both cases he did not lose consciousness. Childhood diseases included whooping cough and measles. He grew with no considerable retardation, and started speaking sentences during his fourth year of age. His sleep, however, was always very disturbed. From the fourth to the sixth year of his life the patient stayed in the Institution for Handicapped Children, where he improved considerably, and the mother was advised to send him to a normal primary school. Although he had to repeat third grade, he later adapted himself and passed from grade to grade, his behavior remaining appropriate.

Since February, 1970, the boy has changed considerably. His behavior deteriorated, he became irritable and prone to fits and, when reprimanded by his mother, he has several times beaten her in the street and thrown things around at home. He began to utter the same word at school, an obscene word which he also wrote in his journal. At times of increased anxiety he would strike his forehead with his hands, making a wry face, blinking his eyelids and uttering inarticulate cries.

In October, 1970, psychological examinations showed mental dullness, although no organic features were found using the Graham-Kendall test for organic features. During his visits to the Children's Psychiatric Dispensary in Katowice, the condition was just the same.

On November 26, 1970, the boy was directed to the Psychiatric Hospital in Lubliniec. When admitted, he was examined, and a white count of 11,800 was found, and the erythrocyte sedimentation rate was 16 mm at 60 seconds. Cerebrospinal fluid was normal. Neurological exam showed asymmetric deep tendon reflexes, with the right side reflexes brisk in both upper and lower extremities. In the conversation with the medical officer of the department, the boy was found to be friendly and easily approached. He was ashamed of his compulsive motor movements, and admitted he is under compulsion when uttering obscenities, particularly when he is cross or "something was not the way I wanted it." "When I failed to do something, I also had to utter a bad word. I struck my head, too, even though it was painful." With startling and vivid emotions he described how he liked to watch television, although at times of tension he would repeat the words, grimace and blink his eyes.

After two weeks in the hospital, a distinct improvement was noticed: his tics were reduced, coprolalia was reduced, and other boys did not irritate him as much. After 21 days of treatment with thioridazine, 25 mg twice a day, calcium bromate, and belladonna alkaloids, the boy was calm, with only mild arm tics and a quiet outcry. The patient was discharged to the Medical Educational Institution where he has stayed to date. Subsequent lab studies show the sedimentation rate at 2 mm per minute and white cell count down to 8500. The electroencephalogram showed some single and serial irregular theta waves primarily in the temporal region.

The second patient, M.L., is a girl born on July 5, 1959, prone to allergic reactions since childhood. Her development was mildly delayed, normal milestones occurring 3 months late. She began school at the normal age and was a good student, although learning was difficult. The malady started with hay fever and a temperature of 37.3°C. When faced with an injection, she became withdrawn, whined, could not sleep and would not obey orders. When admitted to the Psychiatric Hospital in Lubliniec she was found to have an intensely inflamed throat, the tongue was covered with white patches, the sedimentation rate was 14 mm per minute, and urinalysis showed moderate white blood cells. While in the hospital the girl did not make contacts, had to be spoon fed, vomited, could not sleep, did not recognize anyone, and suffered auditory hallucinations. After ten days of treatment with chlorpromazine, 120 mg per day, there was considerable improvement.

Neurological exam revealed increased tonus in the right arm with hyperactive left quadriceps tendon reflex. After 26 days in the hospital, a temperature spike of 37.5°C appeared followed by pain when swallowing.

An otolaryngologist found a subtonsillar abscess and antibiotics were prescribed. The chlorpromazine was discontinued and a return of psychotic symptoms occurred with facial grimacing, arm tics and compulsive barking. When asked by a physician why she did these things she said that she did not know "why I must bark" and "I know that it is not on a level with my age." She is embarrassed, and realizes that her behavior is wrong. The girl also said that in school she "had to bark or cry out," but she did it very quietly and rarely.

The chlorpromazine was prescribed again along with a low vegetative dose of insulin, considerably improving the condition of the patient. She was discharged from the hospital on chlorpromazine, calcium bromate and belladonna alkaloids. She was re-examined as an outpatient two and one half months later and, according to the statements of the girl and her mother, facial grimaces occurred very rarely while all vocal symptoms had ceased altogether. Psychological examination by the Kochs and Arkusz-Bourdon method showed a distinctly increased susceptibility to fatigue and impaired analysis and synthesis of shapes by eyesight, which were likely due to an organic cause.

DISCUSSION

In both of these cases of Gilles de la Tourette's syndrome, the results of examination and the clinical course seem to confirm the organic background of the syndrome. In the case of the boy, the interview suggests prenatal pathology (quinine taken by the mother in the early months of pregnancy). The mental slowness, sedimentation rate, blood count, increased tension of the cerebrospinal fluid and a certain asymmetry of deep tendon reflexes speak for an organic etiology of the syndrome. Also, the results of the interview (home quarrels, abandonment by the father), the neurotic features of the boy's behavior in his early childhood and growing up in institutions for handicapped children must not be ignored and should be listed among the arguments for a psychogenic component of the motor and vocal tics.

In the second case, the interview revealed a long and complicated delivery, delay in the psychophysical development of the child, and a continuous inclination to allergic reactions. The disease started with an increased temperature and psychotic symptoms, and organic features were found in laboratory and psychological examinations. Also, the susceptibility of symptoms to chlorpromazine and insulin treatment indicates as well the organic background of the syndrome.

Continuous follow-up of both patients will be furnishing further arguments.

Gilles de la Tourette's Syndrome. Volume 1: International Registry, p. 123-129, edited by F. Abuzzahab Sr. and F. Anderson. Mason Publishing Co., St. Paul ©1976.

EVOLUTION OF THREE CASES OF GILLES DE LA TOURETTE'S SYNDROME OBSERVED DURING FOUR YEARS

(Comments with Regard to the Social Integration and the Therapy)

J. M. Leger, M.D.

and

Y. Ranty, M.D.

Service de Psychiatrie,
Centre Hospitalier Regional
Limoges, France

Gilles de la Tourette's syndrome was described in the last century after having captivated the medical authorities of that time, but was forsaken for about forty years. Today, it appears that some people are again interested in it, trying to grasp its complicated etiopathogeny and find an effective treatment.

During 1967, in his thesis, one of the authors described four cases of Gilles de la Tourette's syndrome. We were able to examine and interview carefully three of the patients. We were especially interested in the development of these cases on a social basis as well as on the basis of symptoms and treatment since 1966.

CASE REPORTS

The first of these patients, Patrick C., is a twenty-year-old male. His tics began when he was eight years old, some weeks after surgery for a testicular ectopia. He was affected with an intractable hiccup, then with coprolalia directed primarily against his mother. He screamed; exhibited some tics of the face; bit his lips, cheeks and tongue so that he left many scars. In order to prevent nail biting, his hands were covered with rubber gloves. The tics increased to involve the lower limbs and he kicked as if in a temper tantrum.

The boy was violent, savage, unintimidable, and impervious to psychotherapy.

Admitted into a psychiatric hospital, 15 drops of thioproperazine methanesulfonate t.i.d. were prescribed to him, and very quickly we saw a regression of all the symptoms of the disease.

Twice we interviewed this boy. The first time, in 1966, we were presented with an adolescent of middle height, obese for his age, with pleasant manners, answering the questions thoroughly. He appeared to like the medical surroundings and tried to be liked by it, and knew very well his disease and the name by which it was called.

During that interview, which lasted about an hour and a half, no tics occurred. His mother asserted that the symptoms had disappeared after the treatment and admission to the psychiatric hospital. Only the scars on his face gave evidence of the tics' gravity and his self-aggressiveness.

We interviewed this boy again in August, 1970. He appeared to us as in 1966: calm, obedient, and without tics. His parents told us that he left the psychiatric hospital in December, 1966 after which he remained at home only three years.

In February 1968, he again began to become agitated, screaming, jumping and striking his mother with his fists. This situation led to another hospital admission and the symptoms again diminished.

Now he is in the hospital, where he works as a nurse's assistant. He is a boy that appears a little unpolished for his age. He did not progress socially. Since the disease began, at the age of eight, his parents took him from school and had him treated. He was on several occasions admitted to hospitals, and stayed in some for very long periods. Thus, his going to school was interrupted by his parents' initiative and strangely, they refused to send him back to school in spite of the rapid disappearance of the tics after each stay in the hospital. They were afraid that school would trigger a relapse. The patient is currently in good health but lives as an inmate in the psychiatric hospital. The parents are quite unwilling to apprentice him. They still are afraid of a relapse and of the difficulties of adaptation.

The second of these patients, Mr. L., is a 64 year-old male. The syndrome began while he was eight years old, with violent tics of the right limb and of the face, then later with some tics of the right leg. Coprolalia did not appear until then. The disease accelerated his going on a pension and he has not worked for 14 years.

Our first interview with this patient was in 1956. He appeared to us as a man of average height with an alert look, clever, and cultured. His tics were variable and were separated by long periods of time. One must stay at least one hour with him to see one or two tics. When they appeared, however, they did so with extreme violence and were accompanied by a vocal tic, "hem".

He described his coprolalia to us and confessed that often he used to utter some obscene words in church, in open places, in the cinema and also each time he was doing something that bothered him.

Treatment with haloperidol diminished his tics. Although this treatment was effective, he stopped taking his medication quickly, complaining that he was "without reaction and could do nothing."

We saw him again in August, 1970. Always likeable and friendly, he talked to us about his disease and its development. He no longer had coprolalia, possibly because he no longer goes into churches. The motor tics have decreased, and the patient gave us this explanation of his improvement: The tics still occurred when he was doing difficult or very engrossing work, and also when he was idle and someone looks at him. He adds that, when visiting a museum, for example, he will have no tics when alone and free to do what he wants, but when following a guide with several other visitors, he will become irritable and a flood of tics will appear.

He speaks and walks very quickly and although retired he is very brisk. One can feel that he needs activity. Now and then he rises at 3:00 a.m. to work in his garden, he tells us. He is obsessed with work; very meticulous, very scrupulous, stubborn and trusts only in himself. In fact, he built his own house alone, for he has no trust in the professionals.

It appears that he has some sexual obsession. He copulates every day, and sometimes twice a day. When he has no women, he masturbates. He explains this comportment as being absolutely necessary to his health: "It is a spent energy and I feel more relaxed after the sexual act."

When he is working, he never has tics, and an entire day may be spent without agitation.

The third patient, Mr. B.R., is a 54 year-old male. We saw him for the first time in 1965. He appeared to us as a clever man, with good manners, but whose approach inspires at once compassion and dread. He displays a severe case of Tourette's syndrome: Tics of the face, limbs and neck of extreme violence, which brought him a deformation of the face and a traumatic cataract of the right eye. These motor disorders were accompanied by an impulsive and explosive coprolalia.

The patient has been afflicted with this dreadful disease since he was 12 years old. Many people are familiar with him, for he has been quite remarkable. He makes dreadful faces, twists and stretches his neck, hammers his head and belly, screams, utters obscene words, sputters and makes other gestures which are more or less wicked and exhibitionist.

He was always fond of the quarters in the center of town. Thus, in Limoges he frequently took walks in the neighborhood of the railway station where all the inhabitants could see him. They spoke about him, and the children either imitated him or were afraid of him. He was a curiosity which inspired sympathy or repulsion. He gives an impression at once surprising and laughable, but pitiful. He disturbed the public order and on several occasions was summoned and put under restraint of residence.

Thus, since age twelve, he endured frustrations. After family frustrations (his parents were divorced, his mother died when he was young, and his father gave him an unhappy boyhood and never accepted his disease as real) and numerous admissions to hospitals, after numerous treatments without effect, R.B. was to know a new frustration, the social frustration. Society repudiated him.

He left Limoges and began a "French tour," to Bordeaux, Toulouse, Toulon, and Marseilles. In all these cities he was disturbing the peace and was expelled.

What could he do? His mother was dead, his father did not want to see him. The only thing left for him was the confinement from life that he vehemently refused. He decided to go and live in Paris. Curiously, Paris admitted him. "This town admits many others," he once said. Thus for the last 20 years he has lived in Paris, in a quarter of the capital which is particularly animated — Pigalle Square.

There we saw him again in September, 1970. His condition is unchanged; he admitted that he had cut off the therapy prescribed to him while he was in the hospital at Limoges in 1968.

The tradesmen of this quarter, who know him well, told us that sometimes he was calm enough. When an event or a word affected him directly, an explosion and a suite of motor and vocal disturbances appeared and then lasted all day.

DISCUSSION

We have just illustrated three observations of Gilles de la Tourette's syndrome. Two of these cases evolved over many years (one for 56 years, the other for 42 years), the last one for 12 years.

Early authors wrote that the evolution of the syndrome led to madness. At the moment, we can't have the same judgment or the contrary opinion. But it seems hardly imaginable that this "disease of degeneration" leading to madness could have so long an evolution. Moreover, the two patients with lengthy investigation have complete lucidity, can memorize more than the average, are men of sound judgment, have faculties of observation which are absolutely normal, a longing for culture that is sometimes excessive and obsessing; in short, they have all the talents that make clever men out of these patients, certainly not on the way to degradation.

We saw in our three patients that the symptomatic evolution of the tic itself has been very variable over 4 years. The youngest suffers no agitation, and during this period had only one short-lived relapse. The second saw his motor tics in a nearly complete regression since his retirement as long as he has an important physical activity. His vocal tics have practically disappeared. As for R.B., the Parisian patient, his state is unaltered for four years. Motor and vocal tics follow one another all day, with occasional moments of real intermission.

Nearly all authors make a point of describing the tic without giving an interpretation, looking upon it in terms of a motor disorder. One of us showed in a report that Gilles de la Tourette's syndrome had significance. Why does the tic disappear in some patients, regress in others, and why does it persist or increase in some unfortunates?

We showed that Gilles de la Tourette's syndrome should be examined not only through motor pathology but also as tightly connected with the neurotic personality complex of this type of patient. We know that the tic always reproduces a gesture or a mimic, quite particular and distinct from choreic movement.

Wallin[472] makes us notice that there is a difference between the notion of gesture and the notion of movement. Psychomotor motricity is a language. The motor phenomenon in this instance, the tic, is connected with the structure of the psychic life. It is raised to the level of the totality of the person. It is not a simple mechanism of execution, but each stage, each degree of its organization, is the immediate expression of the connections that have settled between the human being and his surroundings. It is in this aspect that we want to look at Tourette's syndrome.

The motor tic, as the observations show, is a means to manifest an aggressiveness. We know that the aggressiveness engenders masochism according to this sequence: The frustration of love engenders the hate, hate engenders aggressiveness, agressiveness engenders the masochism and the provocation engenders the punishment. The punishment, owing to the sadistic response that it constitutes, appeases the need for love and strengthens the hate in justifying it.

We know and we have seen in our patients that there was nearly always a situation of familial conflict: The patient left frustrated.

We said that the tic was a language and that it revealed the connection between it and the surroundings. The first environment in which the child develops is the familial one. In all our patients, it proved to be filled with some conflicts which varied in degree. There was much conflict in the case of R.B., in a lesser degree with L., and still less in P.C.

R.B.'s parents never accepted his disease. Moreover, they frequently quarreled. They were divorced, and the mother died when she was young, and the father took no more interest in his son. He no longer desired to see him, for he was ashamed of him. The patient felt removed from any familial environment, and experienced social frustration.

The lack of regression of his tics, in spite of numerous treatments and hospital admissions, led him to think that medicine was powerless. He consulted some healers, but still without success. He gave up the idea of finding a cure, and began to work — reading medical books, attending lectures, and becoming adept at a naturalist method based on vegetarian diet and hydrotherapy. He obtained, it seems, a good result. But his disease became malignant during the war, for his life was put out of order by the imposed privations.

After the war, he tried to resume his former way of life, but this time fruitlessly. He then understood that his illness was incurable. Having no family and refusing hospital admission, only one route was open to him — vagabondage. He met some oppositions with numerous police actions against him, and this renewed social frustration and the feeling of outcast. One could observe that each time this occurred, his symptoms became worse.

Now R.B. lives in Paris. He eats only ice creams, since different foods exacerbate his symptoms. He sleeps where he can and where he wants, most frequently in the lobbies of the underground railway. Sometimes, when he is restless, he walks all night in the streets of Paris. He has a vagabond's manners, but he wants to continue this way of life. He always vehemently refuses to retire to the country, far from the glances. He wants to live in society and gain acceptance there. Would the loneliness in the country be a form of denial?

Our second patient, L., also spent his childhood in frustration. The tics appeared after a separation from the family circle, and they progressed all his life, with some periods of remission. Initially, his tics were very violent and persisted until adolescence. At this time, they became less intense and less frequent, allowing the patient to marry. His union was a happy one, and he lived comfortably until his retirement.

We can think that this patient found in his wife the love, affection, and understanding that he had not found during childhood.

Unlike R.B., this patient knew no social frustration. He worked as a postal clerk in a provincial small town, and easily became part of his professional surroundings and was accepted by his colleagues, who did not worry much about his tics.

It was the same with our young patient, P.C. He is now in hospital surroundings where he feels well integrated, and his family surrounds him with much love.

We wanted to show, by the description of these three observations, how Tourette's syndrome could perhaps be influenced by the family surroundings and the society. We must note that the patient most affected was the one who, his life long, was the most rejected. The patient the least affected is the one who is now the most accepted.

Thus, the personality of the tiqueur and the evolution of his tics are conditioned by his environment. We share the opinion of Kiever: "The world of adults is not made for the unstable psychomotor. The world of the unstable has neither the coherence, the order, nor the continuity of the world of adults."

The four years of observation also permitted us to reflect on the therapy of Tourette's syndrome. Only one patient accepted the therapy, and he had spectacular regression of symptoms. We must add that, each time, there was an admission into a hospital and isolation from the family surroundings. The other two patients nearly always refused treatment and when they did accept it, they stopped treatment quickly despite having symptomatic relief. We also noticed in both the appearance, paralleled to the psychomotor improvement, of a depressive syndrome. "It is as if someone took the ability to act from me," said one of them. "Activity is necessary to me and it is cut out." The whole problem in the therapy of Gilles de la Tourette's syndrome happens to be summed up in these two sentences.

At the beginning of this affection, the tic is very likely connected with a functional disorder of the motor-integration system, but very soon takes a particular significance, for it takes place in a neurotic personality where the obsessional symptomatology is at the fore.

At the beginning of the illness, it is possible, to some extent, to provoke a regression of the symptomatology thanks to effective chemotherapy with haloperidol and to psychotherapy. But if the patient is seen later, or if the therapeutic conditions have not been fully performed, the disease is going to progress. The motor tic will extend, and the vocal tic will appear with all its significant importance. In most cases, it is of minor importance in the presence of the motor tic. This patient, confronted with the therapeutic failures, will have to accept himself as a man with chronic tics. He will have to modify his world and rebuild a new life through alterations in his personality.

This existence is, in a way, a successful equilibrium of life. To suppress the tic is to ruin this equilibrium; it is to compel the patient to reconstruct a new world, a new life. He must again think over the system of organization of his psychic life modeled since childhood. It is to compel him to put down everything and to begin again.

What will be left to him if this gesture, which becomes a language, is suppressed? Is the patient afflicted with Gilles de la Tourette's syndrome capable of learning another language? We do not think so when the illness is one of long standing, and this is the reason, among others, why it must be necessary to treat these patients soon, before this language of tics is organized and confirmed.

Gilles de la Tourette's Syndrome. Volume 1: International Registry, p. 131-142, edited by F. Abuzzahab Sr. and F. Anderson. Mason Publishing Co., St. Paul © 1976.

PARAVERBAL PSYCHOTHERAPY IN A CASE OF TOURETTE'S DISEASE

Mary C. MacKay, M.D.
Assistant Director, Children's Service,
New York State Psychiatric Institute
New York, NY 10032 U.S.A.

and

Evelyn Phillips Heimlich
Research Assistant, Children's Service,
New York State Psychiatric Institute
New York, NY 10032 U.S.A.

This paper describes the collaborative treatment of an eleven-year-old boy who suffered from Gilles de la Tourette syndrome. During the first of his two years at the New York State Psychiatric Institute, the authors worked separately with him, employing different modalities.

The first author applied the traditional psychotherapeutic approach on an individual basis and also included the boy in some of her sessions with members of the family. (She is responsible for the introductory findings and the summary). The second author employed the paraverbal method in the case. (She reports on the techniques used, selected sessions in this aspect of the treatment, and also pertinent exchanges between the two therapists as to ongoing developments in the case).

Paraverbal therapy is a method of observation and treatment which has been developed at our hospital over a period of fifteen years. It has been particularly useful with children having various kinds of communication difficulties, such as muteness, articular disorders, withdrawal, hyperactivity, and aggressiveness. The treatment of these cases requires that the child's maladaptive behavior be decreased while a therapeutic relationship is developed with him. The goal of paraverbal therapy is purposeful attenuation of those disorganizing affects aroused in some children when exposed to conventional verbal therapy.

What must be understood by the child is stated paraverbally — that is, through rhymes, nonverbal vocalizations, speech cadences, familiar song melodies, and body movement. Such motor activity encompasses the use of miming, percussion and stringed instruments, and drawing to music.

Seven of the 250 children treated with paraverbal therapy, both at the Psychiatric Institute and at a residential school for disturbed and retarded children, suffered from tics. Five of these children improved markedly. Some decrease in uncontrolled movements was observed in the two who remained tiqueurs.

INTRODUCTION TO THE CASE (M.M.)

Billy came to our inpatient service at age eleven years with chief complaints of severe multiple tics and coprolalia. A child neurologist at Columbia-Presbyterian Medical Center had suggested to us the diagnosis of Gilles de la Tourette syndrome based on the above symptoms plus findings associated with minimal brain damage. On psychiatric examination we too arrived at the same diagnosis.

At the time of admission to the hospital, he showed increasing fear that things would get out of control, that if he "let go" there would be terrible consequences. Sudden and loud noises or explosive action made him extraordinarily anxious. He began to have paranoid ideas about hair being in a hole in his mouth. He became preoccupied with thoughts of death. Five months prior to his admission to the hospital, he was withdrawn from school after a virus attack which was followed by a pronounced increase of his symptoms. His parents were particularly disturbed and embarrassed by the appearance of coprolalia which drove them to seek help from their pediatrician. On his advice Billy saw a psychologist who referred him to the Neurological Institute. After examination they in turn referred him to Psychiatric Institute as an inpatient.

Billy was an unwanted child whose mother was ill during the first years of his life. From the start, the patient was a difficult child. When he was one week old and the first time the mother picked him up, he trembled violently and turned blue. He was a hyperactive baby who never seemed to enjoy being cuddled. He was always a feeding problem. Various formulas were tried but to no avail. His preference seemed to be for water, tea or any other liquid. As he grew older his feeding problems continued. When he was started on solid food he did not like it. He was weaned from the bottle at age two.

At a very early age he began to have trouble with constipation. Under the pediatrician's guidance, the mother tried various techniques for helping him move his bowels. These met with but temporary success. By the time Billy was four years old, the struggle took on such proportions that it was decided to have an exploratory operation. When a biopsy of the rectal mucosa was performed, Hirschsprung's disease was ruled out. The parents were told the problem was an emotional one. Gradually they relaxed about the subject and Billy was eventually able to take care of his bowel functioning by himself. With the cessation of this problem motor tics began at about age six, followed by coprolalia at about age nine. Billy did not speak until he was three years old. He became increasingly sensitive to loud noises and to strangers.

From the toddler stage on he slept in his parents bed. One night just prior to admission to the hospital, he called to his mother, after having had a nightmare. He told her it had to do with his having witnessed his parents having sexual intercourse a long time ago. Whenever he remembered this episode, he became terrified. At that time it looked to him as if his father was fighting his mother.

Billy had always been a poorly coordinated youngster. At the time of his admission he had not yet established dominance in either hand, eye or foot, although he used his left hand and foot more than his right, and his right eye more than his left. It was observed that Billy had difficulty in spontaneous expression on any subject that involved his feelings.

Psychological testing did not reveal any striking evidence of thinking disturbance. Although Billy had normal intellectual endowment, he was functioning at a grade two level in school. His reading was markedly below grade level. The tests further showed immaturity with strong oral dependency needs with intensive anxiety and depression stemming from his inability to accept or handle extremely hostile destructive feelings toward parental figures for not satisfying oral needs.

The father, who on the surface was a quiet, easygoing man, had a violent temper and on one occasion even smashed his television set. The paternal grandfather had killed a man in a rage. The mother had a rather hysterical personality with much acting out both in the past and present. When she was a late teenager she had had a fist fight in the middle of the street with her sister over a pair of shoes. Prior to her marriage to Billy's father, the mother had been married to an epileptic of whom she was irrationally frightened when he was in a seizure. She would take a club to bed because she was afraid he would "get out of hand." Ironically he died at the end of a year of marriage while in status. Currently she was often seductive with Billy, competitive with her other child, Bunny, a fifteen-year-old girl, and at constant war with her husband. On occasion she would make threats of suicide.

The family lived in a one-bedroom apartment. Billy shared the bedroom with his sister and the parents slept in the living room. In this cramped and unfortunate situation, one could easily believe with Fenichel[164] that Billy's twitchings were only a form of eroticism representing an equivalent of masturbation. Psychiatrically there seemed enough evidence in the patient's family background to account for a purely functional etiology similar to that in a case described by Ascher:[12] "Most of the symptoms of the disease could be understood in terms of the patient's relationship to authority figures". It was also felt in agreement with Mahler and Rangell,[297] that there were some constitutional considerations as well, which were reducing the patient's ability to withstand "overwhelming emotional and psychodynamic factors."

During the first two months of Billy's stay at Psychiatric Institute, he showed little progress. He was timid with the other children, stammering when they spoke to him and inept at games. At school, he was three grades below his appropriate age level. He did poorly in class, was inattentive, and stammered when questioned. In his individual sessions, references to affect-laden subjects brought only silence or stammering. Family sessions upset him so much that he was excused from them.

Since Billy had such difficulty communicating in traditionally conducted individual and family sessions, it was decided to attempt to get the case moving through the use of paraverbal therapy. This aspect of the case involved fifty-two group sessions (with two other children present) and two individual sessions. His sessions of traditional psychotherapy with Dr. MacKay continued, during the period of his exposure to paraverbal therapy. One of the specific goals of the latter treatment was to help Billy sublimate his erotic and aggressive twitchings.

In the half-hour music sessions, conducted twice a week, Billy was treated with two other children — Lew, eleven years old, and Sue, twelve, who were in treatment for other problems in expression. This report on these sessions is concerned exclusively with Billy's response to the paraverbal method.

The therapists regularly exchanged information gleaned from their respective sessions with Billy. These discussions were mutually helpful to them. Billy revealed different aspects of his personality in his relationship with each of them, not only because of the different treatment modalities employed but also because of the presence of the two other children in the music sessions. The therapists had many opportunities to reinforce each other's interpretations. In each treatment setting, concurrent interpretations were given.

Because Billy responded significantly to the use of the paraverbal method, a detailed description of this aspect of his treatment is presented.

USE OF PARAVERBAL PSYCHOTHERAPY

Instrumental dialogue was improvised by the children and the therapist. The children used primitive percussion instruments such as drums and cymbals, on which they could express themselves without fear of making mistakes. Their rhythmic improvisations were answered by the therapist, usually on the guitar or piano. The children also improvised song accompaniments on the percussion instruments. This was the introductory rhythmic expressive activity at each session.

Projective use of song content: When one of the children was unable to verbalize his feelings on a problem, he was helped to do so through a pertinent song. For example, feelings of rejection were more easily communicated through the song, "Sometimes I Feel Like a Motherless Child." The expressive components of the song (loudness, softness, tempo, accent, etc.) were exploited to the hilt. Usually this technique stimulated the child to comment on his unrevealed feelings. Sometimes, however, the stimulus for verbalization came from a perceptive group member who at that moment could articulate more easily. Comment would then ensue from the child toward whom the song was actually directed. Otherwise, the therapist would ask what the whole song or phrase meant.

The children used percussion instruments to accompany the therapist; on occasion they sang along with her too, imitating her strong affective expression. At times, the songs were spontaneously dramatized by one or more of the children. On occasion, they voluntarily changed the lyrics to suit their current expressive needs. Of prime therapeutic importance were the open-ended questions on song content raised by the therapist. Ensuing discussion of individual problems often produced insight and permitted confrontation, just as the discussion of a dream may. Billy's characteristic silence or denial in early sessions suggested a need for distance, which this approach achieved.

Specific rhythmic expression: Ball bouncing, skipping, jumping, stretching, and song dramatization and miming all to improvised music were geared to further specific motor expression.

Improvisation with chalk and finger paints: Symphonic recordings of markedly rhythmic character, such as Shubert's "Marche Militaire," were played to stimulate the children to create their own designs. They worked at easels to which sheets of paper (20 x 16 inches) were clipped. A wide range of colors in thick pastel chalks and finger paints were available to them.

Revelatory song-stories were improvised and developed by Billy and the therapist in two individual sessions, both conducted in the final phase of treatment. The therapist improvised on the piano, stimulating Billy to verbalize his fantasies. These song stories were sung and played back to him, phrase by phrase, thus further stimulating his expressivity (see session fifty-three below).

CLINICAL APPLICATION[1]

The following material illustrates high points in Billy's development during the course of the fifty-two sessions in which the above-mentioned techniques were employed.

Sessions 1-8: During the early sessions, Billy exhibited shoulder and neck tics as well as coprolalia. Although he showed much pleasure during the rhythmic drum dialogues with peers and therapist, his body movements were extremely rigid. He used only his right hand on the drums. He extended his left hand horizontally, and did not move it. Several weeks passed before this rigidity abated.

When a song was introduced for projective use, he listened carefully to the verbal reaction of the other children. The song "I Used To Love Her But It's All Over Now" evoked heated comments from them on parental fighting and wifely disloyalty. Although these were two areas of acute distress in Billy's home, he remained mute during the discussion. However, he did laugh heartily when Sue and Lew exchanged ideas about fighting behavior of their own parents.

Billy was gradually introduced to more and more types of rhythmic motor activity, such as rhythmic body movement while sitting or standing in one place. He also began to explore and master many primitive percussion instruments and to discover the expressive values of playing soft or loud, fast or slow, according to how he felt.

Session 9: The first "breakthrough" took place at this session in three different areas.

(1) For the first time, Billy showed aggression openly: he threw gobs of finger-paint at his easel. This was done in direct imitation of Sue, who had commented on his inability to put his fingers in the paint-pots. She said encouragingly, "Look, Billy. I throw gobs at the easel first. Then I begin to paint with the music." Laughing, he copied her daring aggressive motions.

(2) In direct imitation of the therapist, he began to use strong, purposeful, expressive motions on the various instruments. As he did so, all signs of his tics disappeared.

(3) Billy for the first time participated voluntarily in the projective use of song content.

---

[1] Pertinent interchanges between Dr. MacKay and Mrs. Heimlich are reported in the bracketed paragraphs included in this section.

It so happened that, just prior to this session, Dr. MacKay, in discussing Billy's psychosexual problems with Mrs. Heimlich, had mentioned that unconsciously he did not know whether he was a girl or a boy and was completely unable to verbalize this uncertainty.

The therapist introduced the song "Rocka My Soul in the Bosom of Abraham" and asked the open-ended question, "What is this song about?" Billy pointed to his own chest and stammered "a woman's these." Sue giggled. Billy, in his first direct reference to his mother, then said, "My mother told me there was once a girl who had a penis." When the therapist remarked that he might have misunderstood his mother or she might have made a mistake, he stammered, "My mother doesn't make mistakes, she brings me up perfect." At this point, Sue produced a confrontation by asking Billy, "If you have such a perfect home life, why are you here?" The question was unanswered. The therapist, rather than pressing further into an anxiety-provoking area, commented briefly that sometimes a mother does too much for her child.

Informed of the content of this session, Dr. MacKay pursued the psychosexual material further in her next session with Billy. He talked freely about his psychosexual confusions.

Session 11: Billy volunteered information on his discussion with Dr. MacKay. When the therapist reintroduced the song "Rocka My Soul" he said, "You did that for me, I mean that part about the bosom. I talked to my doctor about that yesterday and I don't have to giggle about it anymore. But I didn't finish talking about my mother to her." He started to tic when he disclosed more details about his session with Dr. MacKay.

Dr. MacKay, impressed with Billy's progress, had already suggested that it was time for him to try going home for an entire weekend. An experimental visit was permitted. Problems were brought to the fore in the next family session, which was largely devoted to a discussion of the mother's wish to continue having Billy in bed with her. Informing Mrs. Heimlich of the situation, Dr. MacKay suggested that the mother now had to contend with a new Billy, whose more expressive, aggressive, and masculine behavior made her panic. The mother's response to the new situation was to intensify her quarrels with her husband and her daughter. Bunny was unable to cope with the added stress; she, too, had to be hospitalized. All this chaos and anger upset Billy. According to Dr. MacKay, he feared the loss of self-control. He began to display tics again.

Session 12: To provide him with an opportunity to discharge some of his tension appropriately, the therapist involved him in a variety of new and pleasurable rhythmic activities, such as jumping, ball-rolling and bouncing, and two-handed bongo drumming. He responded enthusiastically, playing so loudly that he drowned out the other children. While so expressing himself, he displayed no tics. Billy also enjoyed projecting his ideas on the content of a song on marital friction, "I Wish I Was Single Again." He became so talkative that the therapist had to intervene to provide Lew and Sue with opportunities to express themselves.

Session 21: In the directly preceding sessions, Billy had talked freely about family quarrels, but had not been able to express himself on his relationship to his mother. On this account, the therapist began to sing the lullaby, "Sleep, My Little One." Interrupting her, Billy asked "Could we do a lullaby that my mother always sings to me?" (This was the first time he had shown sufficient verbal independence to do what his peers had often done: request a particular song). He started to sing Brahm's "Lullaby" and the therapist joined him. It was observed, however, that his accompaniment was strikingly inappropriate to the song. Instead of using tender delicate strokes, Billy played the autoharp loudly and violently.

When informed of Billy's inappropriate accompaniment to the lullaby, Dr. MacKay suggested that Billy was ambivalent toward his mother. He still longed for his mother's tenderness, yet her overprotective attitudes angered him.

So overwhelming was his anxiety after singing this song that discussion of its content was postponed to a more propitious moment. He was moved into a new form of rhythmic locomotor expression, *i.e.* rhythmic jumping to accented music improvised by the therapist. He keenly engaged in this activity and left the room looking relaxed.

Sessions 22-28: During these sessions, Billy regularly requested his mother's lullaby. At one session it helped him verbalize his anger at being babied by his family as well as to discuss his sister's jealousy. At another session, he became agitated when singing the lullaby. Instead of confronting him, the therapist put some distance between him and the disturbing song content by deliberately asking the other boy in the group how he felt about the lullaby. Lew said, "It's about a nightmare and somebody trying to hurt me with a whip." Billy, interrupting him, said "Yes, the child has nightmares. He thinks the mother had terrible troubles with the father and the father fights the mother and beats her up and the mother tries to make the child feel better with the lullaby." Then, Billy turned to the therapist and said, "Please, let's do that lullaby again." But this time, his accompaniment was appropriate. Instead of being violent, it was flowing, soft, and tender.

When the nightmare interpretation of the lullaby was reported to Dr. MacKay, she remarked that it might be a reflection of the anxiety aroused in Billy by recent discussions of violence in the family sessions. In one session it was mentioned that the father had hurled a television set across the room in the mother's direction. Billy, who was now attending these family sessions, listened in great agitation to reports of family quarrels. He was silent throughout.

At this time, the presence of his hospitalized sister and her therapist at the family sessions confronted Billy with a new challenge, to which he responded with a certain amount of poise. Dr. MacKay attributed his new increased stability to his favorable interaction with Sue in the music group. Billy now seemed to regard her as a kind of a substitute sibling.

Session 48: After learning about Billy's inarticulateness at a family session at which the father reported a serious suicidal attempt on the mother's part, the therapist introduced a pertinent projective song, "The Midnight Special." This song of sadness and anger stimulated Billy to talk about his feeling of guilt towards his mother, and also of his waning fear of his father. The boy said, "I used to be afraid of him because he was yelling all the time, but now I know that yelling is just a part of him. And now I know that he isn't going to do anything terrible when he uses a loud voice. It's just the way he acts when he is angry."

Billy's increased ability to express himself appropriately was apparent. His bodily movements were now purposeful and without rigidity or jerks. He spoke without stammer or tic on such formerly anxiety-provoking subjects as hostility toward parents, family quarrels, sex differences, and obscenity.

Session 53: Billy was now ready for a more sophisticated form of combined verbal and music expression: the song-story dialogue. One was produced in this one-to-one session to music improvised by the therapist.

First, after stimulating him with a musical phrase played rapidly and loudly on a low register of the piano, she said, "This part is the father." Then as she played a phrase in the middle register, she said, "This part is the mother." Next, playing a phrase on an upper register, she asked, "Who is that?" He said, "Those are the children," and plunged into a story of anger in an imagined family.

"Well, once upon a time there was a father and he was not a good father and he was yelling at the mother and the mother got so excited that she was yelling at the children." He paused. To stimulate Billy further, the therapist played and sang back his words fortissimo, accenting the words, "yelling." She played in two-four march time.

He went on: "Then the father slapped the mother and the mother killed the father and the children were crying." When Billy paused, the therapist again played and sang back his words, this time strongly accenting "slapped" and "killed." "That's good," the boy said and continued. "Then after the mother ran away to Mexico with the children and stayed there for the rest of their lives, and the children got to hate the mother so much that they left her there forever. They grew up and then they went to New York again and there were three girls and boys in the family and they got a job in New York."

After improvising softly to this part of the story, the therapist asked, "What did the boys do?" Billy continued, "One boy had a job in an office and the other boy he worked in a gas station and one of the three girls got a job as a secretary and the other girl got a job in a candy store and the other girl got a job in a lunch wagon — no, make it a restaurant."

To match this part of the story, the therapist improvised music in three-quarter time, playing it in a calm, flowing manner. Billy then said, "Well, that's all there is to the story."

Informed of the song-story, Dr. MacKay said that Billy was still inarticulate, both in the family and individual sessions, on the subject of his parents. Yet the story confirmed his new attitude toward them.

PATIENT'S SUBSEQUENT DEVELOPMENT (M.M.)

At the end of Billy's first year at the New York State Psychiatric Institute, a staff meeting was held for a detailed review of his case. Specifically, it was noted that the boy's favorable response to paraverbal therapy sessions was carrying over into his other activities. Although there was continuing evidence of neurophysiological immaturity, in general, his functioning was much improved. Dr. MacKay reported that she was now able to do some meaningful psychotherapy with him, particularly in the area of his ambivalent feelings toward his parents and his jealousy of his sister. Other staff members commented on Billy's growing ability to make use of milieu, occupational, and recreational therapies. It was recommended that he attend a regular school in the neighborhood, and that he join a local recreational center.

Intensive work was continued with the family, and when Billy left the Institute at the end of his second year, an attempt was made to have him remain at home. This did not prove feasible, however, because of the degree of pathology in the parents. He was then placed in a cottage-type residential setting, where he remained symptom-free. During his stay there, he picked up an extra grade at school, and won awards in painting and sports.

At the time of the last follow-up visit, made four years after his discharge from the hospital, Billy had just returned home. Then sixteen years old, he was in his age-appropriate grade at his neighborhood high school. With his parents and sister, who had continued to get some help in the interim, he appeared to get along well. He had reasonably good relationships with his peers. He was symptom-free except for a recent anxiety attack before his first date with a girl. A referral was made locally for some supportive psychotherapy.

DISCUSSION

From a survey of the literature one is impressed with the fact that the treatment of Gilles de la Tourette's syndrome is a difficult and uncertain one. The chief emphasis has usually been on the control of the symptoms, where drugs have usually been the treatment of choice.

In this case we decided to use the symptom itself in our treatment. Moreover, since this case was being treated under a research program in paraverbal therapy, we decided to forego the use of drugs. Otherwise, it would have been impossible to determine whether the results achieved in the case were due to medication or the paraverbal intervention. We reasoned that since Billy's verbal and motor tics had developed after his constipation problems had been cleared up, we were merely to remove with drugs or psychotherapy the current symptoms which were apparently a defense against aggressive and/or erotic feelings, the patient would be forced to devise a more formidable defense. Instead, we would make an effort with the paraverbal method to harness the presenting symptoms, to channelize the uncontrolled muscular movement into expressive purposeful rhythmic avenues. In addition, with the decreased anxiety thus experienced during the course of such treatment, the patient would be given the opportunity gradually to verbalize and deal with some of the psychogenic aspects of his illness.

One aspect of our rationale in Billy's treatment stemmed from Margaret Mahler's[300] observations that, in treating the tic syncrome, "it is essential to facilitate channelization of the increased amorphous motor urge. Performance activity of the small as well as the large muscles of the body is useful, and, wherever possible, artistic outlets should be encouraged."

A review of the case suggests that both organic and psychogenic factors were implicated in the pathology and had a mutually reciprocal influence. The fact that Billy was not a cuddly baby and turned blue at one week when his mother first picked him up may well have compounded her already rejecting attitude towards him. She had resented her pregnancy from the start. Then there was Billy's persistent fear of bodily contact as well as his hyperactivity. Both made it difficult for him to accept the nurturing he needed and craved. This deprivation could easily have produced in him the rage and guilt so clearly revealed in his psychological tests as well as in his ensuing sessions when he became able to express himself. That he lacked spontaneity and did not speak until age three could indeed have been an additional source of overpowering frustration to him. His long-felt inability to express his distress at his witnessing of the primal scene must have been a further contribution to his tension and tics. That all this took place in an acting-out family who had learned from its history to fear expression was an additional repressive burden for Billy. His life circumstances put him in a double bind. His experiences were such as to produce overwhelming rage. Unfortunately, they took place in a framework of such extraordinary control and repression that normal channels for expression were closed to him. The tics ensued. It was to help Billy cope with these untenable circumstances that we introduced him to the therapeutic approach described. The fact that a follow-up of the case has revealed consistent remission of the tics as well as satisfactory integration of the patient into society makes us feel that this approach merits report. Using our theoretical assumptions and observations it appears the paraverbal method of communication was helpful.

As Billy became more completely involved in many kinds of rhythmic activity one could observe a gradual decrease, then total cessation of bodily tics. Bodily expression was purposeful. He could at will express anger, joy, sadness, or whatever else he had in mind: sometimes as he developed mastery over his movements, their meaning became vividly apparent. At times, he emphasized his meaning by simultaneously verbalizing what he expressed bodily. Sometimes he used percussive accompaniment to underscore the content of folk songs or improvised rhymes.

It is our intent to continue to investigate the use of the reported method with other Gilles de la Tourette patients.

SUMMARY

The treatment of an eleven-year-old boy with Gilles de la Tourette's syndrome at the New York State Psychiatric Institute is described. The two authors collaborated in the case. The report focuses on the clinical use of paraverbal psychotherapy, introduced as an additional therapeutic modality when the boy failed to respond adequately to conventional psychotherapy. Several techniques employed in group and individual music sessions are described, and the use of the components of music as a tool for bodily as well as verbal expression is illustrated.

The use of the paraverbal method in a case of Gilles de la Tourette's syndrome are delineated. This mode of communication permitted the young patient to maintain a therapeutic distance from the therapist, and the erotic elements of music were effectively exploited to help him sublimate his aggressive as well as his erotic twitchings. Through this unorthodox approach, a youngster with severe handicaps in verbal and motor expression became accessible within a year to conventional psychotherapy and to other modes of treatment available to him, including the traditional milieu, occupational, and recreational therapies.

Gilles de la Tourette's Syndrome. Volume 1: International Registry, p. 143-149, edited by F. Abuzzahab Sr. and F. Anderson. Mason Publishing Co., St. Paul ©1976.

GILLES DE LA TOURETTE'S SYNDROME: REPORT OF FOUR CASES WITH EXTENDED FOLLOW-UP

Doris H. Milman, M.D.
Department of Pediatrics,
State University of New York,
Downstate Medical Center,
Brooklyn, NY 11203 U.S.A.

The disorder of multiple tic, described in 1885 by Gilles de la Tourette,[198] although uncommon, continues to attract considerable clinical attention because of its dramatic symptomatology and its disabling social consequences.[167] Still unresolved is the question of etiology and whether multiple tic is a syndrome or a disease.[285] There are good arguments for an organic cause[106] and persuasive evidence for a psychogenic etiology.[167] The fact that its onset is most usually in childhood lends support to the proposition that it is a developmental disorder related to the more benign form of childhood tic.[102] Lacking a proven etiology, treatment remains symptomatic.[94] Recent experience with chlorpromazine[276] and haloperidol[176] indicates that pharmacotherapy can be highly effective even in the absence of a better definition of cause.

CASE REPORT

Case 1

B.B. was first reported on in 1960.[324] He was a white boy of American Jewish background. His symptoms appeared at the age of seven years, with head and body movements that were first diagnosed as Sydenham's chorea. Over the next two years his symptoms progressed to include bizarre body movements, involuntary vocalizations, and coprolalia, resulting in withdrawal from school. The past history revealed hyperkinesis, headbanging, and rocking in early childhood. He came from an intact family without any significant psychopathology.

B. was markedly underweight, owing to the excessive caloric expenditure necessitated by his ceaseless tic activity. The electroencephalogram was normal. Intelligence was in the average range with indications of a higher potential. Projective psychological test data pointed in the direction of neurotic development.

Beginning at age nine, B. was treated with psychotherapy and amphetamine drugs. He was free of tics at the age of 11 years, 10 months. He remained free of symptoms through the completion of high school. At age 18 he entered the army and was cleared for classified work.

Now, at the age of 30, he has been steadily employed in a managerial position since finishing his army service seven years ago. He is married and the father of two children. He is free of psychiatric symptoms. He is virtually free of tics except for "very mild" ones, inapparent to outsiders, when he is under stress.

Case 2.

M.S., a white boy of American Jewish background, was first seen at the age of 9 years, 1 month, because of multiple tics of two years' duration. At the onset of his symptoms, at the age of 7 years, he was thought to have had chorea although he had no fever and no impairment of speech or handwriting. He developed in succession eye-blinking, head-nodding, tongue thrusting, snorting, shrill screaming, and compulsive verbalizations. His parents described him as disobedient, self-willed, sensitive, and unusually fearful. He was afraid of school, new places, doctors, dentists, dogs, injections, and injury.

He was the older of two children in an intact family. Birth, development, and medical history were unremarkable.

Psychiatric examination revealed an unusually immature, dependent boy. His intelligence was in the average range. He was obsessively preoccupied with his body and had many bizarre ideas about its function and malfunction. All of his fears centered about the possibility of bodily injury. There were indications of confusion of psychosexual identification. The diagnosis was personality disorder with hypochondriasis and passive-aggressive elements.

Psychotherapy was undertaken with the primary aim of enabling M. to rationalize and neutralize his anxiety. As he got older his fears became elaborate and included fear of attack by strangers as well as fear of mutilation or body dysfunction. The tics fluctuated in intrusiveness, the most troublesome being the shrill cry, coprolalia, and a heaving motion of the abdomen.

A variety of medications was employed including meprobamate, trifluoperazine, prochlorperazine, diphenhydramine, and diazepam. There was no clear evidence that any of these affected his course.

The tics improved gradually but he remained phobic and hypochondriacal. He was always able to maintain himself in school and his academic progress was satisfactory. Therapy was terminated at age 13 years, 3 months, when he was able to control his tics in public and had gained a relative mastery over his fears.

He remained stable until age 16, when his mother died suddenly of an acute myocardial infarction and his father developed carcinoma of the prostate. M. then experienced a major exacerbation of body anxiety and hypochondriasis, his concern being focused chiefly on his heart. Despite the stress, however, he remained free of tics. He is now 17 years, 6 months, a senior in high school, and planning to attend college.

Case 3.

S.G., a white girl of American Jewish origin, was first seen at the age of 8 years, 3 months because of a vocal tic (*i.e.*, "grunting sound") of three months' duration. For the previous two years she had exhibited a variety of tics and mannerisms, chiefly hand and arm movements and, while eating, a thrusting of her fork toward her eye. Her symptoms started a few months after her parents were divorced. Her mother characterized S. as high-strung, self-willed, sensitive, and generous.

S. was the older of two children. Her relationship toward her brother was ambivalent, with much rivalry, bickering, and resentment. She was clingy, possessive, and demanding toward her mother. She maintained close contact with her father, step-mother, and baby half-sister of whom she was very fond. Her mother had remarried and she had a wary, distant, sparring relationship with her step-father.

On initial psychiatric evaluation S. was found to be of average intelligence. Her thinking was clear and logical. Vocal and facial tics were manifest only in the presence of her mother. Her chief defenses were denial and avoidance. When challenged she regressed readily into helplessness and clinging dependency. The diagnosis was reactive disorder with tics, passive-aggressive and regressive trends.

Initially she was seen at infrequent intervals for consultation and medication. There were fluctuations in her symptoms with periods of improvement and exacerbation. One year and four months after the original consultation, at age 9 years, 7 months, psychotherapy was undertaken because of worsening of the tics and involuntary obscene verbalizations in the classroom. Therapy, consisting of support, ventilation, and interpretation, was continued for 9 months, then discontinued on the parents' initiative because the symptoms fluctuated as before, apparently independent either of psychotherapeutic or environmental events.

Throughout the period of observation a variety of medications was employed successively: Hydroxyzine, prochlorperazine, haloperidol, and meprobamate. No sustained improvement was obtained with any of these drugs. When the parents terminated psychotherapy, they also discontinued all medication.

The present status, at age 11 years, 9 months, is that she still has tics which fluctuate in degree. The movements that bother the mother most are thrusting her fork toward her eye and "spreading her legs." She also has a verbal tic which sounds like "fucka" and which the mother finds "very embarrassing." However, S. is able to control her behavior in school and suppress the tics. Her adjustment otherwise is described as "very normal." Her school work is very satisfactory. She recently had a traumatic experience in the sudden death of her father's second wife. She showed no increase in tics and has assumed a very motherly attitude toward her father and her half-sister. The parents are accepting of the situation and are not seeking treatment at this time.

Case 4.

S.F. was first seen at the age of 15 years, 3 months because of multiple tics, involuntary vocalizations, and compulsive verbalizations. His symptoms reportedly started at the age of 13, at the time when his grandmother, who resided with the family, was dying of cancer. His adjustment was said to have been normal until the onset of the tics; thereafter he became increasingly solitary and his school work deteriorated.

He was the older of two children of an intact family of American Jewish origin. His younger brother was diagnosed as having minimal cerebral dysfunction and low normal intelligence. A paternal uncle was diagnosed as having chronic schizophrenia.

Psychiatric examination revealed a small, slender adolescent boy with facial acne and a variety of facial and body mannerisms and tics. He vocalized a frequent explosive "hah", "him", or "fu" sound. His intelligence was average to high average. On a superficial level he was relevant, coherent, logical and conventional in his thinking. Projective material, however, showed incongruities, bizarreness, pre-occupation with wrong-doing and punishment, poor judgment, and poor reality testing. There was great body anxiety, homosexual anxiety, and guilt over masturbation. His chief defenses were obsessive-compulsive mechanisms, rigidity, and avoidance. There were strong indications of an underlying schizophrenic process.

His symptoms worsened over the ensuing two years to the point where he was smashing windows and bruising his face with self-inflicted blows. He was unable to attend school or go out in public because of his uncontrollable coprolalia. Psychotherapy with another psychiatrist was ineffective. At 18 years he was hospitalized and treated* with large doses of haloperidol and then with fluphenazine, both without effect. In fact, his tics became more extreme and took the form of touching his father's genitals and his mother's breasts and exposing himself. At age 18 years, 6 months, he is being treated with combination of diphenylhydantoin, haloperidol, and phenobarbital plus intensive psychotherapy. On this regimen he is relatively free of tics and free of agitation for the first time in five years, and is completing high school.

DISCUSSION

These cases conform to the experience of others[167 243] in respect to age of onset (predominantly before 10 years) and sex (ratio of males to females of 3:1). They also coincide with the general experience in having normal intelligence and a relatively favorable outcome[167 243] (Table 1).

The question of etiology, unresolved elsewhere, is not appreciably illuminated by this small series. In cases 2 and 4 traumatic events preceded the development of tics, but in the other two cases there were no antecedent events. Moreover, the major psychological trauma that case 3 experienced with the death of his mother did not reactivate his tics. The three boys exhibited similar kinds of psychodynamics, namely body anxiety and sexual anxiety. These are problems that are related to age, sex, and the developmental process and are not specific for any psychiatric disorder. In fact, they are often encountered in boys with no psychiatric disease.

With respect to organicity, these cases do not resolve the issue. Case 1 had an early history that is sometimes associated with minimal brain dysfunction. He had no confirmatory finding in later childhood, however, and became a completely normal adult. Cases 2 and 3 presented no

* At Hillside Hospital under the care of Dr. Jochanan Weisenfreund.

TABLE 1

Case No.	Age at onset	Age at starting therapy	Evidences of organicity	Psychodynamics	Psychiatric diagnosis	Medication	Outcome
1. B.B. male	6 years	9 years	hyperactivity in early childhood normal EEG	fear of bodily injury xenophobia	neurotic traits	amphetamines	free of tics at 12 years good adult adjustment with virtual freedom from tics at age 30
2. M.S. male	7 years	9 years	none	fear of bodily injury Confusion of psychosexual identification xenophobia	personality disorder, passive-aggressive type	meprobamate trifluoperazine prochlorperzine diphenhydramine diazepam	tics controlled at 13 years free of tics at 17 years
3. S.G. female	6 years	9 years	none	dependency	reactive disorder — neurotic traits	hydroxyzine prochlorperazine haloperidol diazepam	tics partially controlled (*i.e.* in public) at age 12 years
4. S.F. male	13 years	15 years	none Family history of psychopathology and organicity	fear of bodily injury xenophobia homosexual anxiety masturbatory guilt	schizophrenic disorder	haloperidol fluophenazine diphenylhydantoin phenobarbital	progressive worsening and deterioration hospitalized at 18 years and showing slight improvement

evidences of organicity. Case 4 had a positive family history that included instances of minimal cerebral dysfunction and schizophrenia. The patient himself, however, had no organic stigmata although he did have a schizophrenic-like illness.

The outcome with respect to control of tics was excellent in two cases, satisfactory in one, and poor in one. The favorable results appeared to be related to the combined use of medication and psychotherapy. No opportunity was allowed for the possibility of a spontaneous remission in adolescence, as has been reported,[167] since the three who improved were treated in childhood. The one patient who did poorly differed from the others in several important respects: he was the only one with a post-pubertal onset; he had a family history of psychopathology; he had an underlying major mental disorder; and he was unable to develop a sustained psychotherapeutic relationship.

This group of patients cannot be used to demonstrate the relative efficacy of one drug over another. The variety of drugs employed testifies to the fact that no one drug was of clear benefit. Haloperidol[419] which appears to be so effective in so many reported experiences, was of only temporary value in these cases. Diazepam was effective in controlling anxiety even when it did not affect the tics per se.

In conclusion it can be re-affirmed that the syndrome of Gilles de la Tourette is a symptom-complex which can be associated with a variety of psychiatric disorders and which is amenable to whatever treatment is appropriate to the underlying disorder.

SUMMARY

1. Four cases of multiple tic of Gilles de la Tourette are described, of whom three were male. Three occurred in middle childhood and one in adolescence.
2. The outcome was favorable in three and poor in one. Stability was maintained over a period of two to 18 years despite both the ordinary and extraordinary vicissitudes of life.
3. A poor outcome was associated with adolescent onset and major underlying psychopathology.

Gilles de la Tourette's Syndrome. Volume 1: International Registry, p. 151-157, edited by F. Abuzzahab Sr. and F. Anderson. Mason Publishing Co., St. Paul ©1976.

GILLES DE LA TOURETTE'S SYNDROME: A CASE REPORT

Libuse Richterova, M.D.
Prague 5, Kartouzska 14
Czechoslovakia

The patient, Frantisek K., was born February 22, 1952, and has been under treatment since March 19, 1962, when he was 10 years old.

His father, born in 1923, is a skilled worker and heavy drinker who has had several problems with his drinking habits. The mother, born in 1924, is a workwoman who has undergone treatment for neurotic difficulties in a psychiatric hospital. She has a simple personality and is emotionally labile and anxious. Her father was an alcoholic.

The mother was pregnant only once. The patient's birth was premature (8 months term) and complicated by a 2-kg (4.4 lb) birth weight, a few minutes of asphyxia, and rather grave icterus neonatorum with dyspepsia until the age of 4 months. He slept little and cried a lot. Growth and development were retarded, as he began to sit up at age 12 months, began to babble at 3 years, and did not speak distinctly until the age of six. His pre-school years included chicken-pox, whooping-cough, tonsillitis, and Asian flu. He was re-trained from a left- to a right-hander. At school age he suffered from parotitis, and in 1962 (age 10) underwent surgery for bilateral cryptorchism. He was ascertained to have a disorder of speech and sight and glasses were prescribed. He has always been sensitive, sorrowful, timid, and tearful.

Data on upbringing are unreliable. The mother said at one time that he had stayed with his paternal grandmother until 2 years of age, and at another time that he had lived with her and his father in an environment of conflict until 3 or 4 years of age (the parents were divorced in 1955 when the child was 3). After the divorce, she handed him over to her own mother, who was living in the country and behaved queerly, subsequently being hospitalized. The boy stayed with this grandmother for 3 years. Subsequently, following a local doctor's advice, the mother placed her son in an unrelated family, where he was brought up by an 81 year-old woman whose grandson (a disabled man 6 years younger than the mother) has been on intimate terms with the mother. At the time the boy was first examined, the mother was thinking of marriage, as her son took a fancy to this man and called him "Daddy." During the mother's visits, the boy behaved rudely or indifferently, and his "foster mother" complained of his disobedience and lack of discipline. He appeared to be unmanageable. He has never been friendly with his classmates, and they scoffed at him for what they called his "hoot," which was taken to be a bad habit he had acquired from his foster mother, who suffered from compulsive coughing and uttered the sound "mnhm."

He started attending school at the age of 6, and got along well save for complaints about his conduct ("he does what he likes"). He suffered from disturbed sleep, and slept little.

After the operation for cryptorchism in 1962, his behavior strikingly worsened. His mother ascribed this to narcosis, and the school doctor referred him for psychiatric examination "for an educational problem — inappropriate response and psychomotor restlessness." The boy was attending the fourth class of the basic nine-year school curriculum at that time. The school mistress reported that "he interferes with others by uttering sounds during a complete silence. Last summer it involved stubborn coughing of nervous origin. He is cruel and exasperates his classmates. He behaves decently towards teachers, and from time to time he works faultlessly. He does well when given additional instruction. He is recalcitrant in nature, hardly manageable, unbending. His lack of discipline has worsened. He has a speech disorder and utters sounds and shrieks inappropriately and attracts public attention."

During this time, the boy was living with his foster mother and future stepfather. They occupied a one-room dwelling and had no belongings, and the mother just called on them. She observed restlessness in her son, with twitching of the mouth and face, compulsive fidgeting with the fingers, and hand-wringing. This display excited the mother, and she became angry and assumed that he did it on purpose and deserved punishment. She admitted that otherwise the boy had good points: Besides being compliant, he was ready to go shopping and was obedient if treated gently.

Results of the first examination (March 19, 1962):

The boy appeared passive, uneasy, and spoke in a low voice. Occasional grimaces and sounds were observed, as well as a disorder of speech characterized by stammering and stuttering. Gait, writing, and drawing were without abnormalities. He complained of having difficulty at school: "The schoolmaster is angry with me. My way of behaving gets him excited." The boy uttered low-voiced sounds like alternate coughing and whimpering. He mentioned spontaneously that he would like to get rid of them. According to his allegations, these sounds have lasted two years and were learned from his "grandmother" (*i.e.*, foster mother), with whom he has been living. He claimed to like going to school and to have good friends. He likes sledding and hockey.

Physical examination revealed asthenia and deep tendon hyperreflexia. Other findings were normal. Intelligence was average, with a score on the verbal scale of the Wechsler Intelligence Scale for Children (WISC) of 96.

Good rapport was established, and psychotherapy was initiated with a session every two weeks. He was given meprobamate, 200 mg t.i.d.

The foster mother and her son (the patient's future stepfather) were invited to the next examination, but they did not come. During psychotherapy, the patient reported that he did not have any dreams. He wants to have a fine, light, lovely apartment and to lose his tic "so that I won't be ruled out from society after I have grown up. I would like to become an engineer so as to be able to invent convenient, speedy, but economical motors. I wish I was a fabulous old man who could satisfy people's desires, and a television so that I might be of use to the one who buys me."

Reports from school testified to a favorable change in his behavior, his tic being limited to an occasional sniff. The patient related that his improvement is due to living with his mother in a proper apartment, and that he is getting along well with his stepfather.

In October of 1962, the mother considered further treatment unnecessary, and felt that the boy's situation at home and at school was good. During the interview the boy's tic did not occur, although when he is left alone he occasionally utters low-voiced sounds (''noyohm'').

The mother appeared with the boy a year later. Her statements were again unreliable. She reported that he had been without any difficulty since before the summer holiday, and then complained that there was no improvement in the boy's state. According to reports at school, he uttered shrieks, shouted both at school and in the street, ''miaow, hello, noyo, sure, cuckoo,'' and whistled. People took it for provocation.

The mother responded to the patient's behavior with anxiety, and when it was discussed, she felt sorry for him and cried in his presence. The schoolmaster threatened him with poor marks for misbehavior and informed us that ''the boy is obstinate, cruel, rude, moody, and hostile.'' The boy expressed the desire to be sent for treatment ''to unlearn it,'' and the mother also insisted on treatment, saying that tenants of their house complained about the patient and considered his behavior provocative. He was referred for hospitalization.

His first admission was at the children's ward of the psychiatric hospital in Prague in 1964 (February through July). At that time he uttered intense sounds just like a peacock's call and grimaced. He liked being in the hospital, didn't long for home, and his condition was worse every time he returned from home.

The electroencephalogram (EEG) at this time was slightly abnormal, with a great amount of beta waves over the front quadrants, sometimes with right predominance and other times with left predominance. Sporadic sharp waves of rapid alpha order accompanied an unevenness of cortex actions with impressive fast components. A repeat trace after medication revealed no change.

Insulin therapy up to 52 units gave a temporary favorable effect, as did chlorprothizene. Thioridazine hydrochloride and phenobarbital gave no effect. At this time an overfixation on the doctor was noticed.

Further outpatient therapy was recommended at discharge, but the mother ignored this suggestion and didn't return until the boy's state became much worse. The boy screamed loudly and verbally attacked his mother, calling her ''slut.''

At the end of the holiday in 1964 (age 12) he was hospitalized again, looking sullen and mute. He presented with an expressive tic in the masticatory and mimic muscles, yawning, compulsive stretching, and choreic movements of the upper limbs. At intervals of 1 to 3 minutes, loud screams were accompanied by convulsive tics of the facial muscles and a torsion movement throughout the trunk. He had lost weight and revealed a terrified facial expression.

Therapy consisted of subcomatose insulin and levomepromazine maleate. His mood improved, and the patient was less disturbed during his stay, although occasional inappropriate behavior was observed, *i.e.*, he offered to take dishes to the kitchen but carried them away to the dissecting room. Also, he often hoarded the soiled linen of other patients. Echolalia was evident as he often repeated the last word of what he had just heard. His state changed for the better after meprobamate was prescribed, but the facial tics were not affected.

Subjectively perceptible was some deterioration of intelligence.

In November he was discharged with the diagnosis of Gilles de la Tourette's syndrome and suspected incipient schizophrenic disorder. He should have followed an outpatient therapy schedule, but again the mother considered further treatment useless. The school insisted upon further hospitalization for this unmanageable child, as he would shout, call outrageous names, fleer, and echo his teacher's words. At home, he was found running around his room after having been horrified out of his sleep by his own screams.

In the same month he was again hospitalized. Laboratory tests of blood and urine were negative. His EEG's (total of five) were slightly abnormal, with large numbers of theta waves of relatively high amplitude, impressive as groups of spikes prevalent over the central area and front quadrants, and sharp alpha waves. There was an irritant component over the frontocentral areas.

The psychological examination revealed an intelligence in the low average range, below average motor performance, disturbance of concentration, anxiety and uncertainty. He evidenced facial tics, the loud uttering of barking sounds, cramps of the mimic muscles, and repeated movements of the upper limbs. He was occasionally mute, sometimes echolalic, coprolalic, with short series of barking and smacking in the meantime.

His condition improved after psychotherapy and chemotherapy with chlorprothizene and levomepromazine maleate. He should have been given these drugs at home as well, but the mother neglected it. After three months hospitalization, only a slight tic remained: Sniffing and smacking. His behavior was ruder but manageable.

The mother wàs not able to follow the doctor's suggestions and didn't stop rebuking the boy, whose state worsened in her presence. He was even corporally punished. In 1965 he was hospitalized in the children's psychiatric hospital in Oparany, mainly because of coprolalic outcries. In the hospital his condition initially deteriorated, with barking, hooting, cuckooing, and soliloquizing. Later some amelioration enabled him to go home for short visits, but this resulted in worsening. Later on, with the establishment of cooperation with the family, the actual character of the disorder was made clear to both the mother and stepfather, resulting in his discharge in 1967 (age 15). He was maintained on bromisovalum and meprobamate. At this time, permanent degeneration was manifest in his behavior: He was solitary, shy, puzzled. Neurovegetative dystonia and hyperdydrosis were also developing. The EEG was quite normal.

On outpatient examinations in 1967 the mother appeared tense and ambivalent-to-hostile towards the patient. The patient appeared as an introvert with marked depression, transient irritation, and aggressive tendencies. He demanded medication ("for depression") in a threatening manner, and screamed, trembled, and cried. He refused to discuss his difficulty, as he only wanted medications. The mother conveyed privately that the patient was clandestinely taking something, but it could not be discovered where he would obtain drugs or what they were like. He no longer suffered from tics.

On February 9, 1968 at the age of 16, he had an epileptic paroxysm for the first time, while undressing in the evening. He fell down and was unconscious for a while. He had eaten strong cocoa for supper that evening. Attacks then occurred at about 5-day intervals, with no treatment initially. Only after he fell in the street did a passing doctor diagnose grand mal epilepsy and transfer him to a hospital, where an EEG, among other procedures, was carried out. Findings were said to confirm epilepsy. In spite of medication he had further attacks, but less intense and frequent. He had his last attack exactly a year after the first attack. He has not observed any regimen, having felt well since. He should take primidone and diphenylhydontoin, but he disliked them and often skipped his prescription. He has trusted in nobody but the doctor who treated him earlier in the psychiatric hospital, continuing to correspond with him by phone or mail about twice a year.

On February 28, 1970, the patient was asked to come in with his mother. He behaved somewhat negativistically, and was more communicative in his mother's presence. Still, he was reserved, passive, and unresponsive to emotional stimulation. They both alleged that he had been without any difficulties, taking antiepileptic drugs regularly.

At this visit, the patient recapitulated the course of his disorder rather inaccurately and evasively. He asserted that he had no difficulty until 11 years of age, when suddenly there occurred "an automatic twitch and sounds" without any preceding or incidental feelings. When he became absorbed in something, which he hadn't managed to do before his stay in the hospital, the tic would stop for four hours or more. He took a fancy to the doctor he had last seen. The mother visited him regularly and also called on the family of a woman assistant in the hospital who had shown motherly concern for the boy.

The mother stated that he had been taken ill "after having been operated on for cryptorchism between the ages of 12 and 13 years and owing to narcosis and hormonal treatment." At first he jerked with the head and growled, spoke vulgarly in an automatic way, and cried in a shrill voice "as a dog howls — it could be heard far away." He hiccupped, hooted, cuckooed, and was the worse between 12 and 13 years of age, being "awfully bad, he uttered awful outcries, really too vulgar." She said his stepfather was to blame for having ignored him, although he longed for a father. Now, after being talked to by a doctor, they have been getting along well together.

He has never been good at manual work. In the hospital he had been interested in being a locksmith, and entered the trade as an apprentice, but was mocked for being slow. Because of this and his later attacks as well, he often stayed away from work. Because of his frequent absence he never finally completed his training. After the attacks diminished, he took a job at the post office, where he has been quite content.

The mother now spoke about the boy with understanding. The patient himself has been more amenable to establishing rapport in her presence.

He has been solitary, not liking to go out, and has refused to see a doctor and to take drugs. He likes to read technical literature on radio and television electronics, but has no other interests.

The asthenic, internal, and neurological findings are normal. His speech is rapid and difficult to understand, and he speaks in a low, monotonous voice. His mimic responses are insipid, with no other abnormalities.

SUMMARY

The following pathogenic influences were ascertained in the case of a young male patient with Gilles de la Tourette's syndrome: (1) heredity (alcoholism, psychosis), (2) perinatal impairment of the cerebrasthenic type, (3) emotional deprivation, and (4) relevant psychotrauma. The first examination was at 10 years, the disorder having manifested itself at about 8 years and initially having been taken as a "bad habit" acquired from foster mother.

At the onset of treatment, the tic was thought to be of neurotic origin. The typical symptoms (chiefly vocalizations) increased subsequently and as a result his family and school associates assumed intolerant attitudes. The condition culminated at 12 years with echolalia, coprolalia, grimacing, bizarre sounds, and bizarre behavior in social intercourse. From 1964 to 1967 the patient was hospitalized most of the time, remaining in the hospital the last two years to complete treatment and schooling in a favorable environment. Since 1966, no medication has been taken, with no more tics occurring. After discharge from the hospital he responded anxiously due to difficult adaptation, with a transient tendency to pharmacophagia.

For one year, from February 9, 1968, to February 9, 1969, the patient suffered epileptic paroxysms of the grand mal type at 5-day intervals, and was given antiepileptic treatment, which he no longer takes. He has been well since.

Objective findings: Character deviation of an autistic type (likely to be secondary, *i.e.*, deprivation syndrome) and slight neurotic symptoms, suspected on the basis of cerebrasthenia, which would confirm the occurrence of epilepsy.

Organic and psychogenic causes played an undoubted role. It can be assumed that the symptomatology varied with the pathogenesis and therefore a different therapeutic approach (psychotherapy and psychopharmacology) was required during the diverse phases.

Gilles de la Tourette's Syndrome. Volume 1: International Registry, p. 159-162, edited by F. Abuzzahab Sr. and F. Anderson. Mason Publishing Co., St. Paul ©1976.

A CASE OF GILLES DE LA TOURETTE'S DISEASE AFTER 10 YEARS' TREATMENT WITH HALOPERIDOL (R.1625)

Jean — N. Seignot, M.D.
32, Boulevard LaFayette
62-Calais, France

This disease is rarely observed, but is not entirely exceptional; in 20 years' psychiatric practice I have only met two cases, both absolutely typical. The first was in a young girl about 20 years old, who came to consult me about 15 years ago. Administration of the neuroleptic medicines available in France at that time produced no improvement. Unfortunately, I was unable to trace this patient later on to apply a course of haloperidol.

The second case was that of a man, at present aged 45. The tics started when he was about ten years old; they were sharp sideway jerks of the head, accompanied by an inarticulate cry, which persisted for several years. Then, in 1940, after a stay in the country, the boy's tics ceased. The boy, an only child of normal intelligence, passed his primary school certificate and took a course in accounting.

When he was 18, he started work as an assistant accountant and the tics recurred, rapidly becoming more complex. Each time he would utter one or several cries, accompanied by awful facial contortions and sudden violent movements. He would in particular take hold of his ears and tug hard on them or hit his face with his fists as hard as he could. He broke several teeth and subsequently several dentures.

For fifteen years he was treated with all types of sedatives, neuroleptics and tranquilizers, without the least improvement.

In 1957 he underwent a topectomy. The tics disappeared for a few days following the operation but soon returned, as often and as intense as before neurosurgery.

In 1958 his punching and his trying to claw out his eyes resulted in total blindness after intra-ocular hemorrhage and detachment of the retina.

I had promised the patient, who had consulted me in 1957 after the failure of the topectomy, that I would let him know if I heard of the discovery of a new drug offering a possibility, however slight, of helping him. When haloperidol was commercialized in France in 1960, I therefore contacted him at once.

In November of 1960 he was in a particularly sorry state. Not only had he become blind, but his tics occurred on the average of once or twice a minute, each tic lasting about four seconds, during which time he kept hitting his head and trunk and throwing himself about all over the place. The coprolalia was strongly marked, a mixture of shouts, insults and swearing. He was particularly upset at this time because he was obsessed by some uncontrollable impulse to hit his forehead on the sharp edges of furniture and doors.

The effect of the haloperidol treatment administered at this time was absolutely spectacular. The tics ceased almost entirely from the second day on, recurring only rarely, especially if someone spoke to him about his illness. The initial dose was 1 mg per day. To obtain a more complete result, the dose was increased, but had to be reduced, as the haloperidol brought about great lassitude. Finally, with a dose of 0.6 mg per day, taken permanently, the patient had only a few tics a day and no longer experienced the feeling of lassitude.

A few years later, however, the tics became more frequent, in spite of the continued treatment of 0.6 mg per day. Other products were tried with no effect. The dose of haloperidol was finally increased to 3 mg per day, and this made the tics disappear completely. This treatment has been continued regularly at this dose for several years, and is perfectly tolerated with the sole addition of chlorhydrate of heptaminol to counteract the feeling of lassitude caused by the quantity of haloperidol.

At present, the patient is in excellent physical condition and of a lively disposition. His blindness unfortunately prevents him from working.

DISCUSSION

As such good results were obtained by haloperidol, no other butyrophenone derivatives were tried in this case. On the other hand, phenothiazine derivatives had been administered with no success. This patient had never been given thioproperazine, which might also be effective in cases of this disease.

The following remarks may be made concerning this case, which is interesting from a therapeutic point of view:

1. Gilles de la Tourette's disease is unrelated to any other, but it seems probable that it is of the same nature as the ordinary tics and twitches so often met in both children and adults. The initial phase is progressive, and in the present case, consisted of 'barking tics', a more troublesome and serious form than the usual tics.

Haloperidol has been shown effective in the treatment of all kinds of tics, with a high percentage of total success, thus coming up to the expectations held after its spectacular action in Gilles de la Tourette's disease.

2. The theory held by many psychiatrists, and in particular by many psychoanalysts, that tics are manifestations to be connected with obsessional neurosis, would seem to be contradicted by this experiment, firstly on the grounds that haloperidol always has a good result on cases of tics. Such a treatment would be ineffective in cases of obsessional neurosis and indeed often aggravate the condition. Secondly, obsessions do indeed occur in the course of Gilles de la Tourette's disease, as in this particular case. However, some time after the tics had disappeared and the patient was sure they would not return, his obsessions ceased, too. Perhaps one might consider that the tics, being phenomena which repeatedly restrict the activity and the liberty of the patient, might themselves bring the patient to an obsessional way of thinking. Conversely, there is no reason to believe that an obsessional thought structure brings about tics and twitches in certain subjects, whether children or adults, nor that the tics may be assimilated to ritual conjuration in obsessional neurosis, in spite of some points common to both symptoms.

SUMMARY

A serious case of Gilles de la Tourette's disease, hitherto resisting all treatment, has been cured for over ten years thanks to continuous treatment by moderate doses of haloperidol (3 mg per day).

Gilles de la Tourette's Syndrome. Volume 1: International Registry, p. 163-166, edited by F. Abuzzahab Sr. and F. Anderson. Mason Publishing Co., St. Paul ©1976.

GILLES DE LA TOURETTE'S IDIOPATHIC SYNDROME: TREATMENT WITH HALOPERIDOL

Vicdan A. Senler, M.D.
Fellow in Child Psychiatry
Child Guidance Clinic, Inc.
Louisville, Kentucky 40223 U.S.A.

In 1885, when Gilles de la Tourette was studying under Charcot at the Salpêtrière in Paris, he published a description of this syndrome which was later named after him. The syndrome is sometimes referred to as "tic convulsive."

The syndrome begins in childhood, usually in children of school age and before puberty. The patients affected with it exhibit an ever-growing repertoire of motor tics that involve not only spasmodic grimacing but also violent stereotyped tics, spasmodic movements of the upper part of the body, finally involving the whole body until tic-like actions are expressed by hopping, skipping, jumping, grinding of the teeth, and other sudden compulsive motor outbursts that, nevertheless, may involve a certain amount of coordination. Compulsive coprolalia that accompanies the muscular tics gives special flavor to the syndrome. They utter swear words or obscenities, usually "four letter words." This may be accompanied also by coughing, barking, spitting. This strange behavior is exhibited spontaneously and unpredictably by the patient. It may be triggered at times by emotional stress.

CASE HISTORY

R.W.S., an eleven-year-old white male, was referred to our Clinic by a local pediatrician with the chief complaint of having multiple tics and mannerisms. His father's comment was that "he grunted and jerked all over as though he was going into a convulsion." He was having difficulty in school, felt that other children didn't like him and called him names. He became tense and seclusive, and made poor grades. His symptoms were getting progressively worse in intensity and frequency since the age of eight.

Developmental History

The history indicates that pregnancy and birth were normal. There was no evidence of birth trauma. He weighed eight pounds and five ounces. He is the second of three children. He has a sister twelve years old and a sister four years of age. During the preschool years he had the usual colds. There was no evidence of any complications.

At the beginning of the first year in school, he experienced a moderate degree of separation anxiety. He was well-adjusted during his second year but suffered from pharyngitis often. At one time he had "strep throat" with a questionable heart murmur. A tonsillectomy was recommended and done. Following the summer of that year, he started complaining of being "sick." During the middle of the night he would crawl out of his bed and cry loudly. A couple of weeks after that he started saying "swear words" under his breath, later out loud, which was apparently uncontrollable. The parents gave as examples, "Shit! Shit! Hell! Hell!" This occurred at home and church also. The parents first talked to him, then whipped him for it and finally ignored him. Still, he continued these utterances, particularly under stressful situations. A couple of months later he started grunting, and then head, neck and shoulder jerks began. Tics of the face at times were followed by blurts of very loud yelling of the first syllable of a word; then decreasing in a pseudo fashion at extremely low tone, from time to time with a break in the middle of a sentence.

The parents began worrying about this and a family doctor was consulted. The child was given hydroxyzine hydrochloride without any improvement. He began coughing and clearing of his throat; the jerking movement of the head and shoulder spread to arm and chest, gradually extending to the right leg. Throat-clearing, coughing and jerking increased in intensity and frequency. He became withdrawn socially, and did not want to go to school. There was no family history of mental illness, epilepsy or tics.

The father was a thirty-six year-old white male. He was described as a stable and responsible person. The mother was a warm and intelligent woman. Seemingly there was a healthy relationship among the family members. However, the mother's only brother and only uncle had histories of sore throats and died of kidney diseases in their early age. The family has a tendency to believe that the mother's side produced ill-health sons.

When the patient was first seen by us, his prominent symptoms were multiple muscular tics, grunting, coughing, and throat-clearing to a severe degree. He also was found to be grossly insecure, withdrawn, and felt rejected by others. However, he expressed his frustrations in not being able to control his jerkings.

Physical Examination

He was average in height, slightly built. Systematic examinations did not reveal any abnormalities. Laboratory examination was within normal limits. Complete neurological examination was negative. Electroencephalogram was read as moderately dysrhythmic without focal abnormalities.

Psychological Examination

Wechsler Intelligence Scale for Children: He obtained bright normal range of intelligence with verbal scale of 121; performance of 103; FS of 114; restricted inner self with marked passive element which would indicate a personality trait disturbance (passive-aggressive, passive-dependent type). He has a tendency to internalize aggressive impulses. His adaptation in interpersonal relationships, especially with authoritative figures, was poor.

Course of Treatment

First, supportive psychotherapy was initiated weekly. Excessive anxiety tension improved; ability to express feelings was much better. Muscular tics and throat-clearing became less intense but continued as usual.

The starting dose of 2 mg haloperidol daily was instituted in April, 1970. The patient showed a great deal of improvement in a two week period. Muscular tics were controlled and throat tics became almost inaudible. The patient's general attitude for socialization became near normal. During the summer months, he learned swimming and joined the games with other children. At the time of this report, eight months after treatment was started, the patient was in the sixth grade making A's and B's. He is still free of muscular tics. However, from time to time, he exhibits difficulty in his relationship with authority, mostly with his mother.

DISCUSSION

This patient presents symptoms considered essential for the diagnosis of Gilles de la Tourette's syndrome; namely, childhood onset, multiple motor tics, vocal tics, and coprolalia. He sought help because of his uncontrollable jerking and behavioral difficulties. The cause of the disorder is still unknown. Positive neurological findings, extremely rare in previous reported cases, were absent in the present case. Tics have been described as a sequel of encephalitis, which could affect the basal ganglia.[59] Organic difficulty as part of the problem has been supported by many authors.[153, 289] However, management of the patient must be broadly based. The authors' speculation about etiology is that probably there is a strong relation between the infection that patient has had (in the present case a streptococcus infection) and his presenting symptomatology. It is possible that psychological characteristics are the secondary effect of the illness. Treatment with haloperidol, giving excellent results, is in accord with the results of other investigators.[53, 284, 419, 441]

SUMMARY

This paper presents an eleven-year-old boy suffering from Gilles de la Tourette's syndrome, who was treated successfully with haloperidol. It is likely that the etiology of the disorder is organic pathology of the central nervous system; apparently psychological difficulties are the secondary effect of the illness.

Gilles de la Tourette's Syndrome. Volume 1: International Registry, p. 169-183, edited by F. Abuzzahab Sr. and F. Anderson. Mason Publishing Co., St. Paul ©1976.

SECTION THREE: CURRENT KNOWLEDGE OF THE SYNDROME

F. S. Abuzzahab Sr., M.D., Ph.D.
Clinical Associate Professor
Departments of Psychiatry, Pharmacology
and Family Practice and Community Health
University of Minnesota
Minneapolis, Minnesota 55455 U.S.A.

and

Floyd O. Anderson, M.D.
Resident in Psychiatry
University of Minnesota
Minneapolis, Minnesota 55455 U.S.A.

> "If I have devoted so much to the symptomatology and the evolution of the malady of convulsive tics, it is because they appeared to me indispensable in the interest of diagnosis. . . . It might seem to you that these precautions are valueless, given the clear physiognomy of this affliction. Don't believe it. Although fifteen years have passed since I isolated this morbid syndrome, the truth remains that this affliction is still very frequently unrecognized."
>
> Gilles de la Tourette, 1899

INTRODUCTION

The previous series of papers contain much important and new data about Gilles de la Tourette's syndrome. Contributions include twenty-nine new case reports and observations on differential diagnosis, treatment, prognosis and etiology. The purpose of this section is to present this new data in light of what is already known about Tourette's syndrome, with enough history to explain its significance in light of the vast amount of speculation accumulated by hundreds of observers over the years.

SUMMARY OF NEW CASE REPORTS

The authors of the papers in the first sections presented 29 case histories of Gilles de la Tourette's syndrome not previously published in the world literature. Of these new case reports, nineteen come from the United States, four from Czechoslovakia, two each from Hong Kong and Poland, and one each from Hungary and the United Kingdom. In addition to these cases, 26 unpublished case reports from the International Registry of Tourette's syndrome were added (See Table 1). This group of 55 new cases of Tourette's syndrome was compared to the 430 published case reports summarized earlier in a review of the literature (see page 71).

TABLE I. DISTRIBUTION OF CASE REPORTS BY NATIONALITY

Country	From this Series	From International Registry	Total
United States	19	18	37
Czechoslovakia	4	5	9
Poland	2		2
Hong Kong	2		2
France		2	2
Hungary	1		1
United Kingdom	1		1
Canada		1	1
Total	29	26	55

Table II shows the results of this comparison.

When the incidence of each symptom of the affliction in the new group of cases is compared to the incidence in the published cases in the review, no significant differences are found.

TABLE II. COMPARISON OF SYMPTOMATOLOGY IN TWO GROUPS OF TOURETTE TIQUEURS

	Incidence	n_i	p_i	p_{oi}*	Difference⁺
Males	44	55	.800	.705	ns
MOTOR SYMPTOMS					
Facial tics	49	55	.891	.922	ns
Arm tics	43	55	.780	.778	ns
Leg tics	35	55	.636	.541	ns
Neck tics	26	55	.473	.528	ns
Echopraxia	6	55	.109	.085	ns
Copropraxia	6	55	.109	.075	ns
VOCAL SYMPTOMS					
Inarticulations	43	55	.780	.652	ns
Coprolalia	37	55	.673	.576	ns
Echolalia and Pallilalia	12	55	.219	.234	ns

*From table, page 74

⁺ Using Chi-square method of data assessment

Despite the many inadequacies of this type of review, it is important to note that the symptomatology of the syndrome is remarkably similar not only across cultures (see page 76), but also for a period of over eighty years. Such findings seem to imply organicity in the etiology of the syndrome (see page 178).

The ages of onset for this group of patients is presented in Table III. It is seen that 37 patients, or 74%, developed symptoms by the age of eight years, and no patients experience symptom onset later than 13 years. This compares favorably with the larger series (see page 75).

TABLE III. AGE AT ONSET OF SYMPTOMS

Age	Number of Patients
0 — 4	3
5 — 6	17
7 — 8	17
9 — 10	6
11 — 12	6
13 — 14	1
N =	50

Psychologic evaluations include intelligence testing in 35 case reports. Of these, 16 are in the "normal" range, 12 are "below normal," and 7 are "above normal." Our experience with the larger series was that a disproportionate number of IQ scores were above average (see page 75).

At least one electroencephalogram was performed on 26 patients. In 15 case reports, at least one abnormal tracing was obtained, for a frequency of 58%. The vast majority of abnormalities were non-localizing, with "generalized dysrhythmia" most commonly observed. This has also been the experience of Wayne, *et al*[508] who evaluated 34 Tourette tiqueurs with at least one encephalogram and concluded that the higher than expected frequency of abnormalities (50%) suggest an organic etiology and that "localization of the disturbance in the nervous system and mechanisms which cause . . . . Tourette's syndrome remain unknown." Lucas[287] summarized 58 cases and found a similar situation. Feild, *et al*[162] analyzed EEG tracings from seven patients at the Mayo Clinic and formulated the statement that the EEG responses cannot be considered as specific for Tourette's syndrome alone. However, they have observed similar tracings in various types of movement disorders considered to be of uncontested psychogenic origin.

In 17 case reports, a distinct precipitating event was reported. Eight of these involved the death of a loved one, birth of a sibling, and other psychotraumatic episodes such as a dog bite. Seven other cases reported a febrile illness preceding the onset of symptoms. These varied from bronchitis and flu to rheumatic fever, with only one case of mumps and no documented encephalitides. The other two cases began after surgery. One patient had a previous episode of encephalitis of unknown etiology, and two others had a history of head trauma. In one case, the mother had taken alcohol and quinine in the second trimester of pregnancy in an effort to induce abortion.

Family dynamics have been implicated as contributing to the development of the malady.[285 145 149] This series of case reports is replete with unfavorable home situations. Eight case reports described one or both parents as being excessively rigid or domineering, four patients came from families broken by separation or divorce, and two patients were unwanted. Frequent quarrelling, strained interpersonal relationships, or generally unfavorable home situations were mentioned in another eight case reports. Evaluation of these figures is probably meaningless due to the many contributors and lack of any type of standardized psychometric data, and is best left to those series of patients seen by a single clinician. In addition, it becomes a difficult problem to differentiate the psychopathology present before the illness becomes manifest from the psychopathology occurring after or as a result of the illness itself.

The same difficulty occurs when evaluating the mental status of the patient himself[420] and again, the concomitant psychopathology is best evaluated by the clinician in his own series of patients. Twenty of the case reports describe some concomitant psychopathology, of which enuresis is the most common. The other findings are not consistent, and will not be dealt with at length here. Abnormalities of growth and development were described in nine cases, including one case of cryptorchism, two of epilepsy, two failures to thrive and one with severe allergies. These findings agree with those in the larger series (see page 75).

The family neuropsychiatric history in this series is reviewed in the following section on etiology.

DIFFERENTIAL DIAGNOSIS

Gilles de la Tourette's syndrome is one of the most distinctive clinical entities when seen in its full-blown symptomatology. The patient with childhood onset of generalized tics and vocalizations, coprolalia and echolalia, presents few problems with differential diagnosis. However, the course of the illness is variable, and at the time of examination, the diagnosis may not be so evident. Gilles de la Tourette stressed differential diagnosis in his papers describing the syndrome[198 199] and warns:

> "The **course** of this illness as far as we have been able to judge in following the description which we have given, is slow and insiduous. Its origin is obscure. Little by little its symptoms evolve at different dates of appearance. The whole follows a regular enough course; however, in giving the individual history of every symptom, we have said that there are moments of exacerbation for every one of them. These exacerbations are variable in duration and intensity. We should add that when the three coexisted — muscular contractions, echolalia and coprolalia — they became exaggerated simultaneously. As opposed to exacerbations, let us place the periods of remission or lull. Under unknown influences which are variable according to the subjects as far as we have been able to judge, the muscular contractions become less frequent and less strong, the obscene words are no more said except at rare intervals, and the echolalia becomes difficult to distinguish. In these intervals, the cure is never totally complete or radical: the illness is dormant, it has not disappeared. Always the muscular contractions remain. It is true they are attenuated but they are also always easy to perceive: they are centered in an arm or often enough they might localize in the face muscles (Obs. I, II, III, V, VII). These calm periods could be somewhat long (Obs. I, one year; Obs. II, five months; Obs. III, three months, etc.), but at a given moment, the procession of symptoms reappears as accentuated as previously until one day when another remission period re-establishes the calm."

The rarity of Tourette's syndrome is undoubtedly a problem in diagnosis, as most physicians have never seen a case and many have not had any formal education about it. The literature contains several bizarre case histories of patients who have consulted scores of physicians without obtaining an accurate diagnosis or an explanation of prognosis, and have been treated with virtually every type of treatment known to psychiatry.[217 328 420] The rarity of the syndrome is not necessarily attested to by the infrequency of case reports.[383]

The diagnosis of the syndrome has traditionally been based on three features of the history and physical examination:

1. Generalized motor tics
2. Onset in childhood
3. One or more vocal tics

Occasionally clinicians do not include vocal tics in their diagnostic criteria, but our review indicates that less than 5% of patients diagnosed as having Gilles de la Tourette's syndrome have no vocal tic.

The motor tics are frequently very severe, causing fractures[4 18] and in one case, retinal detachment and blindness.[156] Coprolalia, considered pathognomonic, is not limited to Tourette's syndrome; neither is copropraxia or the echophenomena. The following differential diagnosis is based on several diagnostic problems found in the literature:

Sydenham's chorea; chorea minor: Gilles de la Tourette[199] emphasized this as the chief diagnostic differentiation for the clinician. Differential characteristics include other manifestations of streptococcal septicemia, preponderance in girls, fever, difference in the characteristics of the dyskinesia, and self-limited clinical course.

Simple Transient Tic of Childhood:[501] Since the majority of Tourette tiqueurs have only a simple tic at the onset of their illness, differentiation from the very common transient tics can be very difficult, and accurate diagnosis may have to wait for the onset of other symptoms. These tics are very seldom multiple and are usually limited to one muscle or muscle group. Many are responsive to psychotherapy and usually disappear by adolescence.

Encephalitides: To list the clinical features of the scores of different types of encephalitis would be tedious and fruitless. Suffice it is to say that the association of encephalitis with Tourette's syndrome is being mentioned more and more in current literature, and evidence is growing in support of an infectious etiology for the syndrome. Although less than 5% of patients in our review suffered from diagnosed or possible encephalitis, recent evidence from Fisarova (see page 89) and Ivan (see page 43) indicate otherwise. Perhaps subclinical or missed encephalitis is responsible for at least some cases of the illness. Although several extrapyramidal symptoms have been reported during the acute stages of many encephalitides, most occur during the convalescent period, and frequently reflect focal pathology. Many syndromes have been described in the literature (postencephalitic Parkinsonism, encephalitis lethargica and Benedek's (klazomania).

Intoxications:[411] Of all toxic disorders, manganese poisoning most closely resembles Tourette's syndrome, often exhibiting choreiform movements. Also present is extrapyramidal rigidity.

Other points in the differential include hysterical and schizophrenic mannerisms,[77 166 473] obsessive-compulsive disorder, mental retardation, focal vascular lesions, essential myoclonus,[182] myoclonic epilepsy, and Huntington's chorea.

TREATMENT AND PROGNOSIS

The prognosis for Gilles de la Tourette's syndrome has changed dramatically since the development of the butyrophenone, haloperidol (see page 77). Although there were several authors who claimed that the syndrome was degenerative, leading to mental deterioration.[11 207 220] Gilles de la Tourette emphasized in his classic treatise that such is not the case:[198]

> The **mental state** is perfectly regular and normal; the subjects have very good reasoning. In no way do their acts resemble those of the insane. They have perfect awareness of their condition; most are very intelligent. In all our patients, the general sensitivity was absolutely normal. As for the physical, moral and mental state of the patient, . . . it is excellent in all respects except, of course, for the disadvantages created by such an abnormal state.

Partly as a result of its unknown etiology and partly because of its socially crippling symptomatology, Tourette patients have been treated with virtually every type of therapy, varying with what was in vogue at the time (see page 77). In Gilles de la Tourette's time, social isolation was the most effective in reducing the symptomatology, with other regimens ineffective or detrimental.[96 405 451] In the first half of the twentieth century, psychotherapy and psychoanalysis, as well as hypnosis, proved to be of only limited value.[1 5 157 211] Recent therapeutic trials of shock therapy, sleep therapy, neurosurgery, psychotherapy, and a host of psychotropic drugs have shown clearly that haloperidol gives consistently better results (see page 77).[11 167 415 419 430]

Controlled studies of Tourette patients treated with haloperidol are available, but data on a large series of patients is not yet available. There are many single-blind studies and accidental discontinuations that speak for the efficacy of the drug.[34 85 105 111 175 176 328] Double-blind studies have been performed on a single patient by Messiha, *et al*[319] and Connell, *et al,*[99] but there is a great need for further controlled study.

ETIOLOGY

> "As to the intimate nature of this affliction, what can we say in the total absence of any given anatomopathologic findings?"
>
> Gilles de la Tourette[198]

Until recently, very few studies have been conducted in an effort to clarify the origins of Gilles de la Tourette's syndrome. But almost every investigator displayed a fascination with the illness and was willing to propose a theory explaining its pathophysiology. Through the years it became apparent that each investigator felt that the cause was to be found within the area of his expertise, and two groups emerged: those who considered that the syndrome was caused by psychogenic factors, mainly psychoanalysts and psychologists, and those who considered the cause to be organic.

Some feel as did S.A.K. Wilson,[488] that "behind all the phenomena (of tic), however diverse they be, lurks a physical predisposition." Gilles de la Tourette[198] himself said, "We can, with assistance from the resources of psychology, try to interpret some symptoms." Many others agree with A.K. Shapiro:[419] "It is likely that the etiology of Gilles de la Tourette's syndrome is organic pathology. Previous belief that the etiology was psychological was caused by failure to demonstrate organic pathology." Morphew and Sim[332] question whether or not it is a good idea to try to find a common etiology for the syndrome at all. Since much new information is presented in the previous papers, we feel it may be valuable to review some theories as to what causes Gilles de la Tourette's syndrome. It is convenient to divide the review into two parts: the psychogenic argument and the organic argument.

THE PSYCHOGENIC ARGUMENT

There are many reasons why the syndrome of Gilles de la Tourette has long been considered to be due at least in part to psychopathology. Our knowledge of the central nervous system is as yet only rudimentary, and to think that one lesion could cause such a varied constellation of symptoms is difficult. Organic pathology any more extensive would likely interfere with other functions of the nervous system. The absence of any localizing signs in the neurological examination and the consistently negative laboratory examinations of the Tourette tiqueur led to the belief, especially in the first decades of the century, that some psychical abnormality was at the root of the etiological question.

Although Gilles de la Tourette clearly and repeatedly stated that the mental status of the tiqueur remained intact and that there was no evidence of any process of degeneration, the popular concensus after 1900 was that mental deterioration ending in psychosis was to be expected. At least partially responsible for this mistaken concept was Guinon,[207] a contemporary of Gilles de la Tourette at the Salpetriere, who presented a series of four patients with Tourette's syndrome who developed either a psychosis or a personality disorder. Later reports mistakenly quote his conclusions as being those of Gilles de la Tourette. The literature includes several other case reports with a similar outcome, but the total number represents a small percentage.[11 45]

Several other characteristics of the syndrome tend to support the theories of psychogenicity. In a significant minority of cases, a psychologically traumatic episode was associated with symptom onset (see page 75). The symptoms themselves are universally observed to vary in frequency and intensity with situational stress, with an occasional exception.[115 281 285] They disappear during sleep and during intense concentration, and can be willfully suppressed for a time. There is no concrete evidence for genetic transmission (see page 75), and there appear to be no abnormalities of birth or growth and development (see page 75). But, by far, the most compelling characteristics are the coprolalia and copropraxia, and to a lesser extent the echophenomena.

Gilles de la Tourette described the coprolalia this way:[198]

> "It is then in a true moral sense that these coprolalic interjections are emitted. There exists at the moment of emission of these coprolalic interjections an irresistible psychic compulsion which pushes the subject to utter these obscene words without discreetness or the least human respect.

Several reports[157] claim that an intense exacerbation of symptoms occurred when references to religion were made, or when the patient even drove past a church. With such inappropriateness a daily occurrence, many patients chose seclusion. Others have developed different defenses. While shopping, one of our patients with a loud barking tic will join other shoppers in craning their necks to look for the source of the bark. A.K. Shapiro[420] contends that use of the toilet for release of symptoms is so frequent in these patients that it is a presumptive indication of Tourette's syndrome.

With the advent of new psychological theory in the twentieth century and the concomitant intensity of interest in the field, it is no surprise that many new hypotheses and treatments were tried with Tourette's syndrome. What is striking about the psychological evaluation and management of these patients, even through the current studies, is that there is very little diagnostic similarity (or agreement) from paper to paper. It is a problem to determine whether the patients differ more than the investigators. Furthermore, the evaluation of the role of psychopathology in Tourette's syndrome is not made easier by concentrating on one diagnostician: in a recent paper summarizing the psychiatric evaluation of 34 Tourette tiqueurs, all seen by the same psychiatrist,[503] only one patient was found to have no mental disorder. In the remainder, diagnoses were so many and varied that summarizing them is difficult and probably valueless.

Bockner[45] states that "the majority of the cases described in the literature have had factors of an obsessive-compulsive neurosis." Although it is one of the most commonly mentioned diagnoses in those cases with psychopathology, our literature search found it mentioned in about ¼ of the case reports (see page 74). Ascher[11] reported that all of the five patients he studied had obsessive personalities. He also found considerable resemblance, particularly in the case of stereotyped mannerisms and speech, between the features of the syndrome and the symptomatology of schizophrenia. Mahler[299] referred to the anal and markedly narcissistic character structures of Tourette tiqueurs. Hollander[226] stated that the illness is characterised by severe ego defects and a narcissistic orientation. Hysterical patterns are noted, however, in cases described by Schneck,[410] and Aimard[5] states that "a typical oedipal situation was exposed," and in another case a castration complex. Hammer[211] found that "(the patient) and his mother were mutually involved in a sado-masochistic relationship in which they would abuse and get abused by each other." Aarons[1] felt as several investigators did, that "involuntary, diffuse muscular activity can serve not only for discharge of aggression but equally as a libidinal indulgence" and that "this disease illustrates further how the erotization of an organ system may cause its dysfunction to such a degree that it serves the id more than it does the ego." Ferenczi[166] believed that tiqueurs of all types are narcissistic and that tics are "stereotyped masturbatory equivalents." In a series of 34 cases seen by Shapiro,[503] 27 had various personality disorders (only one was classified obsessive-compulsive), four suffered behavior disorders of childhood, and two were psychotic.

Another frequently mentioned symptom is inhibition of aggression[419] and several investigators have turned their attention to family dynamics. Ascher[11] found that symptoms of echolalia and coprolalia appeared when the patient developed unacceptable feelings and attitudes toward one or both parents and attempted to suppress them. Dunlap[149] felt that compulsive sounds and movements of the patient he studied were related to feelings of guilt and hostility directed toward authority figures. Bockner,[45] Hollander,[226] MacDonald,[289] and Slap[428] reported a pattern of strict parental domination and a struggle between the suppression and expression of explosive hostility. Finally, Lucas[285] dealt with this pattern in depth in an excellent report and follow-up of 15 cases (see page), and Morphew, *et al*[332] did the same in their series. More study is needed in the area of family dynamics before a conclusion can be made as to its role in the pathogenesis of Tourette's syndrome.

Psychotherapy has been the most frequent approach in the treatment of Tourette's syndrome (see page), and no specific mode has proven to be consistently effective. Every new mode brought promise of success in alleviating most symptoms, but later attempts proved that successes were not consistently reproducible. Nonetheless, psychotherapy plays an integral role in the treatment of the illness today, not in an effort to control the symptoms but as an essential supportive adjunct to chemotherapy.

Psychological testing has played a minor role in the diagnosis and evaluation of the Tourette tiqueur, and controlled studies using psychometric testing are few in the literature. Piotrowski[369] reported that "no significant difference was found between the Rorschach records of the Gilles de la Tourette's group and the records of another group of tic children." On the basis of psychologists' ratings of the WAIS or WISC, Bender-Gestalt, and Rorschach, Shapiro, *et al*[506] conclude that 76.7% of 30 Tourette patients had signs of "mild" or "moderate" organicity. Mahler and Gross[298] conclude that "clinical observation as well as objective psychometrics reveal that the group of children with tic syndrome have a mean IQ of over average." Several other series report a similar trend, and our review showed that the WISC scores of Tourette tiqueurs were slightly, although insignificantly, above average (see page 75).

In conclusion, it can be said that the argument for a psychogenic element in the pathophysiology of Gilles de la Tourette's syndrome is based on the same evidence today that it was in Gilles de la Tourette's time. Little new knowledge has been advanced in support of it, and fewer investigators insist that psychopathology is a major component in the etiology of this strange malady. There is little justification for using psychotherapy as the first line of attack on the symptomatology, and other than the need for supportive psychotherapy, its value is accurately paraphrased by Gilles de la Tourette:[198]

> We can, with assistance from the resources of psychology, try to interpret some symptoms.

THE ORGANICITY ARGUMENT

> "When I incidentally discussed the meaning and significance of tics with Professor Freud, he mentioned that apparently there was an organic factor in question."
>
> Ferenczi[166]

The emphasis on neurology and organic psychiatry at the Salpêtrière greatly influenced the etiological theories of Gilles de la Tourette and the other early investigators who taught and studied there, among these Charcot,[92] Guinon,[207] Salmi,[401] and Catrou.[80] However, their arguments were based more on hypothesis and suspicion than on empirical evidence. Support for an organic etiology became popular again in the fifties and sixties, but only recently has there been any progress in the proof of the suspicion. Perhaps current ideas, like the psychological theories, are only reflecting the trend of the times. However, recent empirical data appears at this point to be more than suggestive.

There is little in the clinical picture of Gilles de la Tourette's syndrome to suggest an organic etiology. One suggestive fact is that over twice as many males as females are affected, and that the age of onset is almost invariably in childhood (see page 73).

The Role of Infectious Disease. The relationship of the syndrome with infectious disease is becoming more and more significant as more data is gathered. Gilles de la Tourette reports:[198]

> Among the subjects who were submitted to our observation, there were three who, since the onset of the syndrome, had acute infections (Obs. III simple sore throat; Obs. IV typhoid or paratyphoid fever; Obs. VI diphtheria). While the fever lasted, it is unquestionable that the muscular contractions decreased much in frequency and in intensity, without disappearing completely. They did not reappear with their ordinary violence until the disappearance of the febrile state.

Several subsequent investigators observed similar variations in symptomatology with febrile illnesses of scattered etiology. Ross[393] observed symptom amelioration with severe scarlet fever and lymphadenitis, and Jolly[237] reported 15 weeks of amelioration during an episode of typhus. Ascher [11] and Walsh[473] reported a similar correlation.

However, a decrease in symptom intensity concomitant with febrile episodes appears now to be the exception rather than the rule. Nylander[345] reported a direct and marked exacerbation in the frequency and intensity of Tourette symptoms in a patient with several febrile episodes. Creak and Guttman[112] reported a marked increase during a puerperal sepsis, and Faux[161] observed the same in a postoperative, febrile tiqueur. Dolmierski,[142] Challas (Pt. #6)[85] Borak (see page 81), Ivan (see page 43) and MacKay (see page 131) reported symptom exacerbation in patients with measles, influenza, small pox vaccination, encephalitis, and other febrile illnesses with an unmistakable correlation.

The foremost investigator in this area has been Fisarova, whose initial report on 10 Tourette tiqueurs showed this pattern of symptom variation quite clearly.[172] In her paper on page 89, she reports three more cases with this pattern.

Lumbar Punctures. The most likely suggestion from these data is that the syndrome is connected in some way with an infection of the CNS, most probably an encephalitis. The many forms and etiologies of encephalitis make definitive diagnosis difficult, and many cases may be subclinical. However, Fisarova's data obtained from lumbar punctures of her patients

TABLE IV. LUMBAR PUNCTURE RESULTS

Author	Patient No.	Results
Ascher		"normal protein, cell count, pressure"
Baker		"normal"
Bing		"inflammatory changes"
Chakraborty	C.S.	"normal"
Dolmierski		"normal" x 2
Dunlap		"normal"
Eisenberg	5	"normal"
Ivan		"negative"
Levy		"negative"
Magowska		"negative"
Prabhakaran		"normal chemistry and VDRL"
Singer		"normal"
Slap		"clear fluid at 170 mm"
Stevens		"normal"

is quite convincing (see page 93). Inflammatory changes were also reported in several patients from her first study.[171] Bing[39] reported similar findings in a single puncture, but other investigators have not, as is shown in Table IV. It is not clear in most reports, however, how thorough the spinal fluid analysis was. It is plain that further analysis of the possibility of an encephalitic etiology must be pursued, with thorough history and more adequate spinal fluid analysis.

Pneumoencephalography. Six investigators report pneumoencephalography in a Tourette tiqueur. Ivan[233] reports a "normal" examination in one patient, but an "abnormal" one in the case report presented earlier (see page 45). Borak (see page 83) found marked hydrocephalic dilatation of the left lateral ventricle, with a slightly dilated third ventricle. Eriksson[158] also reports a dilated left ventricle which was considered to be a congenital malformation. Dolmierski[142] reports two normal examinations in his patient, and E.F.W. Baker reports one normal exam.[15] Bjarsch[41] mentions the fact that a pneumoencephalogram was performed on his patient, but the results were not clearly presented.

In conclusion, it would appear that the value of pneumoencephalography in clarifying the mysteries of Gilles de la Tourette's syndrome is not clear at this point.

Autopsy Findings. Anatomopathologic findings in Tourette's syndrome are sparse in the literature. Bing[39] reports some nonspecific meningitic thickening upon gross examination of the brain. No microscopic examination was performed. De Wulff and van Bogaert,[136] in a 31 year-old patient, found no extrapyramidal lesions and none of the abnormalities found by Balthasar,[18] which include generalized encephalitic changes ("dwarf growth") in the corpus striatum of a 42 year-old patient.

Our registry includes three new autopsy reports which do not conclusively support any previous findings.

Borak reports autopsy findings in a patient who expired two months after a cryothalamotomy was performed (see page 81). His findings were attributed to congenital vasculopathy involving all areas of cortex and the subcortical structures. The case reports in the International Registry include two additional new autopsy reports: R.Y. (contributor: D.H. Rosen): negative, and E.D. (birthdate 10-4-13): no gross abnormalities (microscopic study not done).

Again we find no clear contribution to the argument that Gilles de la Tourette's syndrome has an organic etiology. Of course, conclusive evidence can never be found in a review of the autopsy findings of so few investigators, but, with consistent and thorough reporting and the use of the International Registry, this data can become more than suggestive.

Neurochemical and Neuroanatomical Considerations. There is still much skepticism in many circles that the clinical picture of Gilles de la Tourette's syndrome could be attributed to an organic lesion somewhere in the central nervous system. There is growing support, however, for the possibility that pathology in the extrapyramidal system is responsible for the bizarre symptomatology.

Some investigators[15] produced experimental spasmodic torticollis in monkeys by placing a small lesion in the medial reticular substance of the tegmentum of the midbrain. The experimental torticollis reproduced all of the features of human spasmodic torticollis, including marked accentuation by emotional stress. This latter feature is especially significant in application to Tourette's syndrome, as a similar exacerbation with stress is associated with most symptoms.

Other investigators[77] associated echolalia with lesions of the left temporal lobe, frontal lobes, and corpus striatum, and Schneider[411] reports echolalia and echopraxia in conjunction with carbon monoxide intoxication, cerebrovascular accidents and general paresis. Coprolalia has also been seen in conjunction with some strictly organic pathology in the central nervous system.[444]

In addition, we know that the phenothiazines and butyrophenones are the most satisfactory drugs in the control of Tourette symptomatology. MacDonald[289] has shown that the phenothiazines act on the corpus striatum and Snyder, *et al*[430] showed that haloperidol acted on dopaminergic neurons, which are abundant in the corpus striatum. Snyder has also suggested that an over-activity of dopaminergic neurons may be the pathophysiology of the syndrome. In support of this is the observation of a dyskinesia very similar to Tourette's syndrome in cases of amphetamine intoxication.[308] [344]These observations, as well as those on the gnawing dyskinesia of rats given high doses of amphetamines, may provide an animal model for future studies in this area.

Heredity. Our review of the literature showed in general that there was no genetic factor in the development of Gilles de la Tourette's syndrome (see page 75). However, there are several families in which the incidence of the disease suggests a different situation.

One of Gilles de la Tourette's[198] initial patients had a sister with the same disease. In 1887, Oppenheim[351] reported the family history of a patient with

Tourette's syndrome which showed a dominent inheritance pattern (see Fig. I). Unfortunately, no follow-up was reported on this family, in which a female tiqueur begot four daughters with "the same disease," and three grandchildren with "the same disease."

FIGURE I. OPPENHEIM'S FAMILY TREE

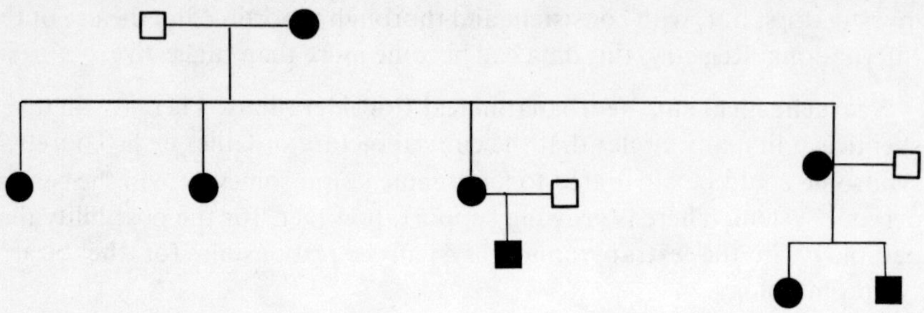

Grafer[202] reported a case whose maternal uncle had the same disease. Feild[162] reported another family history which included three brothers with eye tics and a cousin with questionable Tourette's syndrome. In the International Registry, E.D. (birthdate 10-4-13) and S.D. (birthdate 12-20-47) are father and son, and M.C. (birthdate 5-29-58) is a second cousin of S.N. (birthdate 4-12-58). (Note: Dr. D. G. Sanders at UCLA is preparing a study on the familial aspects of the syndrome at present).

These families represent a very small proportion of the more than 400 reviewed in our series. Five other family histories are replete with simple tics, but the suggestion of a genetic factor ends there. Ellison[154] reports a patient whose monozygotic twin is unaffected. Shapiro[500] reports a patient whose dizygotic twin is unaffected. A larger series of twins is impossible to accumulate since the disease is rare. Follow-up is necessary before any conclusion can be made; but at present, it appears that genetic factors do not play a role in the development of the syndrome.

Cross Cultural Analysis. The analysis of a large series of Tourette tiqueurs has shown that the syndrome is surprisingly uniform not only between samples but also across cultures (see pages 75 and 170). Such uniformity would typify an organic lesion and also tends to speak against a psychogenic phenomenon.

THE INTERNATIONAL REGISTRY

For many years Gilles de la Tourette's syndrome has remained one of the most intriguing of the neuro-psychiatric syndromes, and it promises to remain as such for some time to come. Its rarity has long been used by many as a reason not to invest much time or ingenuity to its etiology and treatment. However, its rarity has been overestimated by most physicians who are not familiar with it, and rare syndromes have often provided clues to the lesser known bodily functions.

In Tourette's syndrome we may find a link between the motor systems and the vast unknowns of the "higher" "cortical" functions, as well as contributions to our knowledge of the biogenic amines, neuroanatomy and behavior.

But by far the most important consideration when investigating this illness is the patient. Gilles de la Tourette's syndrome is a terrible, unrelenting social crippler, which can become the primary focus in the life of one who is unfortunate enough to be afflicted by it. Although the anti-psychotic tranquilizers have shown considerable therapeutic value, the treatment is difficult and frequently inadequate, and no cure is known.

It is with these considerations in mind that the International Registry of Gilles de la Tourette's syndrome was established at the University of Minnesota. The registry has as its primary function the collection and tabulation of case histories of patients afflicted with the illness. All reports are confidential and data are used to enhance the knowledge of many aspects of the syndrome, as well as provide adequate means for long-term follow-up.

Inquiries should be addressed to:

Faruk S. Abuzzahab Sr., M.D., Ph.D., Box 393 Mayo, University of Minnesota Hospitals, Minneapolis, Minnesota 55455, U.S.A.

SECTION FOUR: BIBLIOGRAPHY

REFERENCES

1. Aarons, A.Z. 1958. Notes on a case of maladie des tics. *Psychoanal. Quart.* 27:194-204.

2. Aberle, D.F. 1952. Arctic hysteria and latah in Mongolia. *Trans. N.Y. Acad. Sci.* 14:291-297.

3. Abuzzahab, F.S. 1970. Some uses of haloperidol in the treatment of psychiatric conditions. *Psychosomatics* 2:188-193.

4. Abuzzahab, F.S. and Ehlen, K.J. 1971. The clinical picture and management of Gilles de la Tourette's syndrome. *Child Psychiat. Human Devel.* 2:14-25.

5. Aimard, P. and Kohler, C. 1961. Resultats de la cure de sommeil associee a la psychotherapie dans 10 cas de maladie de Gilles de la Tourette. *Rev. Neuropsychiat. Infant.* 9:110-122.

6. Albrecht, H. 1949. Uber die Ticersheinungen im Kindesalter. *Nervenarzt* 20:314-320.

7. Albrecht, H. 1952. Motorische Unruhe im Kindesalter. *Z. Kinderpsychiat.* 19:145-189.

8. Alexander, L. 1965. Clinical experiences with hypnosis in psychiatric therapy. *Amer. J. clin. Hypnos.* 7:190-205.

9. Andre, G. 1891. Une observation de maladie des tics convulsifs avec onomatomanie. *Mercredi Med.* 11:325-326.

10. Ascher, E. 1949. Motor attitudes and psychotherapy. *Psychosom. Med.* 2:228-234.

11. Ascher, E. 1948. Psychodynamic considerations in Gilles de la Tourette's disease (maladie des tics). *Amer. J. Psychiat.* 105:267-276.

12. Ascher, E. 1966. Motor syndromes of functional or undetermined origin. In *American Handbook of Psychiatry,* ed. S. Arieti, New York: Basic Books, v. 3, ch. 10.

13. Ayd, F.J. 1967. A clinical appraisal of haloperidol. Lippincott's *Med. Sci.* 18:55-58.

14. Bagge, L. and Kalling, M. 1964. (Gilles de la Tourette's Syndrome.) *Lakartidning* 61:3174-3184. Swedish.

REFERENCES

15. Baker, E.F.W. 1962. Gilles de la Tourette's syndrome treated by bimedial frontal leucotomy. *Canadian Med. ss. J.* 86:746-747.

16. Bakwin, H. and Bakwin, R.M. 1960. *Clinical Management of Behavior Disorders in Children.* Philadelphia: W.B. Saunders Co. pp. 430-432.

17. Balducci, M. and Frascella, G. 1962. Un caso di malattia di Gilles de la Tourette trattato con haloperidol (R-1625). *Symposium Internazionale sull'haloperidol e triperidol.* Milan. pp. 177-180.

18. Balthasar, J. 1956-7. Uber das anatomische substrat der generalisierten Tic-Krankheit (maladie des tics, Gilles de la Tourette). *Arch. Psychiat. Nervenkr.* 195:531-549.

19. Barrett, B.H. 1962. Reduction in the rate of multiple tics by free operant conditioning methods. *J. nerv. ment. Dis.* 135:187-195.

20. Barsky, P. 1967. A clinical variant of tic convulsif. *J. Pediat.* 71:417-419.

21. Bass, M.H. 1919. A case of phonation tic. *Trans. N.Y. Acad. Med.* 36:184.

22. Battistelli, L. 1896. Contributo allo studio dei tic convulsivi. *Rif. Med.* 12:746, 759, 770.

23. Beard, G.M. 1878. Remarks upon jumpers, or jumping Frenchmen. *J. nerv. ment. Dis.* 5:525-526.

24. Beard, G.M. 1880. Experiments with the "jumpers" or "jumping Frenchmen" of Maine. *J. nerv. ment. Dis.* 7:487-490.

25. Beer, B. 1898. Zur Behandlung des Tic convulsif. *Wien. Med.* 21:423,440,455,473,489.

26. Bender, L. 1956. *Psychopathology of children with organic brain disorders.* Springfield, Ill.: Thomas.

27. Bender, L. and Schilder, P. 1941. Mannerisms as organic motility syndrome (paracortical disturbances). *Confin. Neurol.* 3:321-330.

28. Benedek, L. 1925. Zwangsmassiges Schreien in Anfallen als postencephalitische Hyperkinese. *Z. ges. Neurol. Psychiat.* 98:17-26.

29. Bennett. 1889. Jumpers. *Lancet* 2:579.

REFERENCES

30. Bergonzini, C. 1891. Tic convulsivo e paramioclono multiplo. *Rass. ital. Ch. Med.* 6:2-34.

31. Berillon. 1903. Maladie des tics convulsifs traitee avec succes par la suggestion hypnotique. *Rev. Hypn. Psychol. Physiol.* 18:377-378.

32. Bernardou, H. 1923. Tics et maladies mentales. *Rev. neurol.* 2:20-27.

33. Bhargava, K.P. and Srivastava, R.K. 1965. Central effects of haloperidol on somatic reflexes. *Brit. J. Pharmacol.* 25:751-757.

34. Bieren, R.E. 1969. Tourette's disease, successful treatment. *J.S.C. med. Ass.* 65:7-8.

35. Bilikiewicz, T. 1957. *Psychiatria Kliniczna*, Warszawa: Panstwowy Zaklad Wydawn Lekarskich.

36. Bilikiewicz, T. 1961. *Psychiatria Kliniczna*, Warszawa: Panstwowy Zaklad Wydawn Lekarskich.

37. Bilikiewicz, T. 1969. *Psychiatria Kliniczna*, Warszawa: Panstwowy Zaklad Wydawn Lekarskich.

38. Bing, R. 1952. *Lehrbuch der Nervenkrankheiten.* Basel: Schwabe.

39. Bing, R. 1925. Uber lokale muskelspasmen und Tics. *Schweiz. med. Wschr.* 55:993-1000.

40. Bixby, E. W., Jr. 1970. Haloperidol for the Gilles de la Tourette's syndrome. *J. Amer. med. Ass.* 211:663.

41. Bjarsch, H. 1972. Beitrag zur Problematik der Touretteschen Krankheit. *Nervenarzt* 43:94-97.

42. Blandin, J., Bonhoure, J. and Soucachet, P. 1961. l'Association tofranil-haloperidol dans le traitement des syndromes schizophreniques. *Ann. Med.-psychol.* 119:988.

43. Blatt, A. 1964. *Rhythmic responsiveness of normal elementary school children.* Ann Arbor, Michigan: University Microfilms, Inc.

44. Bloch, S. 1960. *Contribution a l'etude de la maladie de Gilles de la Tourette.* These, Strasbourg Universite Faculte de Medecine, no. 60.

45. Bockner, S. 1959. Gilles de la Tourette's disease. *J. ment. Sci.* 105:1078-1081.

REFERENCES

46. Boekhoudt, H.B. and van der Weyde, A.J. 1893. Maladie des tics convulsifs. *Nederl. T. Geneesk.* 29 part 2:369-378.

47. Boenheim, C. 1930. Uber den tic im kindesalter. *Klin. Wschr.* 9:2005-2011.

48. Boheimer, W. 1893. *Uber zwei Falle von ausgehartetem tic convulsif.* Bonn.

49. Bojanovski, J. and Nahunek, K. 1962. Gilles de la Tourettuv syndrom. *Cs. Psychiat.* 58:50-52.

50. Bollea, G. and Strazzeri, F. 1955. Il problema nosografico dei tic in base ad uno studio catamnestico. *Infanz. anorm.* 11:137-145.

51. Boncour, G.P. 1910. Les tic chez l'ecolier et leur interpretation. *Progres Med.* 36:495.

52. Borak, W. 1969. Przypadek encefalopatii z tikami Tourette'a zespolem anankastycznym i impulsywymi tendencjami do samouszkodzen. *Psychiat. Pol.* 3:111-114.

53. Boris, M. 1968. Gilles de la Tourette's syndrome: remission with haloperidol. *J. Amer. med. Ass.* 205:648-649.

54. Boschi, E. 1967. Considerazioni sulla malattia di Gilles de la Tourette Contributo clinico. *Arch. Psicol. Neurol. Psichiat.* 38:141-160.

55. Bourneville, P. and Poulard. 1903. Un cas de maladie des tics; guerison. *Arch. Neurol.* (Paris) 16:208-216.

56. Bouteille, E.M. 1810. *Traite de la choree ou danse de St. Guy.* Paris: Vincard, pp. 329:362.

57. Bradnan, W.A. 1972. Familial communicational patterns of a patient with Gilles de la Tourette's syndrome. *J. nerv. ment. Dis.* 154:60-68.

58. Brain, W.R. 1928. The treatment of tic. *Lancet* 1:1295-6.

59. Brain, W.R. 1962. *Disease of the Nervous System, 6th ed.* New York: Oxford University Press.

60. Breitmann, G. 1888. *Contribution a l'etude de la coprolalie, de l'echolalie at de l'imitation des gestes chez les degeneres et alienes.* These de Paris.

REFERENCES

61. Brescia, M.A. 1938. Tics in childhood. *Arch Pediat.* 55:703-709.

62. Bresler, L. 1896. Beitrag zur Lehre von der Maladie des Tics convulsifs (mimische Krampfneurose). *Neurol. Cbl.* 21:965-972.

63. Bridger, W.H. 1962. Sensory discrimination and autonomic function in the newborn. *J. Amer. Acad. Child Psychiat.* 1:77.

64. Brissaud, E. 1896. La choree variable de degeneres. *Rev. neurol.* 4:417-431.

65. Brissaud, E. 1890. Le spasme saltatoire dans ses rapports avec l'hysterie. *Arch. Gen. Med.* 2:385-399, 547-560.

66. Brissaud, E. 1899. Choree variable. *Presse med.* 1:73-74.

67. British Medical Journal. 1962. Children's tics. *Brit. med J.* 5309:903-4.

68. Brown, E.E. 1957. Tics secondary to sinusitis. *Arch. Pediat.* 74:39-46.

69. Bruch, H. and Thum, L.C. 1968. Maladie des tics and maternal psychosis. *J. nerv. ment. Dis.* 146:446-456.

70. Bruetsch, L. Occlusive rheumatic arthritis in the brain and other organs in patients with valvular heart diseases. *Proc. IV, Int. Cong. Neuropat.* 3:309-319.

71. Burot, M. 1887-8. Un cas de la maladie des tics convulsifs traite et ameliore par la persuasion. *Rev. Hypn. Psychol. Physiol.* 2:141-144.

72. Buss, O. 1886. Beitrag zur Lehre von der Aetiologie des Tic convulsif. *Neurol. Cbl.* 8:313-316.

73. Bychowski. 1910. Chlopiec dotkniety choroba tikow. *Neurol. Pol.* 1:101-103.

74. Cainer, A. 1889. Un caso di tic convulsivo con coprolalia. *Gazz. Osp. Clin.* 10:74-75.

75. Caprini, G., and Melotti, V. 1961. Un grave sindrome ticcosa guarita con haloperidol. *Riv. Sper. Freniat.* 85:191-196.

76. Caretto, R. and Barbano, C. 1909. Sopra un caso di malattia dei tics di natura epilettica. *Pediatria* 7:121-128.

REFERENCES

77. Carluccio, C., Sours, J.A. and Kolb, L.C. 1964. Psychodynamics of echo-reactions. *Arch. gen Psychiat.* 10:623-629.

78. Casares, Gil y. 1904. Tic impulsivo y simulacion en una nina. *Cong. int. Med.* 14:972-977.

79. Catalano, A. 1946. Malattia dei tics convulsivi con coprolalia ed impulsi a mordere de trauma cranico o da encefalite epidemica. *Arch. Psicol. Neurol. Psichiat.* 7:367-378.

80. Catrou, J. 1890. *Etude sur la maladie des tics convulsifs (jumping, latah, myriachit).* These, Paris: Henri Jouve.

81. Chabbert, L. 1893. De la maladie des tics (tics, choree, hysterie: diagnostic). *Arch. neurol.* (Paris) 25:10-41.

82. Chakraborty, A. 1962. Gilles de la Tourette's disease. *Indian J. Psychiat.* 4:187-189, 1962.

83. Chakraborty, A. 1968. Gilles de la Tourette's syndrome. *Brit. J. Psychiat.* 114:123-125, 1968.

84. Challas, G. and Brauer, W. 1963. Tourette's disease: relief of symptoms with R. 1625. *Amer. J. Psychiat.* 120:283-284.

85. Challas, G., Chapel, J.L. and Jenkins, R.L. 1967. Tourette's disease: control of symptoms and its clinical course. *Int. J. Neuropsychiat.* 3(suppl#1):96-109.

86. Chapel, J.L. 1966. Gilles de la Tourette's disease, the past and the present. *Canadian psychiat. Ass. J.* 11:324-329.

87. Chapel, J.L. 1970. Latah, myriachit and jumpers revisited. *N.Y. St. J. Med.* 70:2201-2204.

88. Chapel, J.L., Brown, N. and Jenkins, R.L. 1964. Tourette's disease: symptomatic relief with haloperidol. *Amer. J. Psychiat.* 121:608-610.

89. Chapman, A.H., Pilkey, L., and Gibbons, M.J. 1958. A psychosomatic study of eight children with Sydenham's chorea. *Pediatrics.* 21:582-595.

90. Charcot, J. 1886. Hysterie et tics:diagnostic. *Sem. Med.* (Paris) 6:125.

91. Charcot, J. 1885. Intorno ad alcuni casi di tic convulsivo con copralia ed ecolalia. *Rif. Med.* 2:814.

REFERENCES

92. Charcot. J. 1888-1889. *Lecon du mardi a Salpetriere.* Paris:E.Lecrosnier & Bache, pp. 49,60,123,150,209,249,388; pp. 13,463.

93. Charcot, J. 1889. Des tics et des ticqueurs. *Ann. Med. Chir.* 5:1-5.

94. Clark, D.F. 1966. Behaviour therapy of Gilles de la Tourette's syndrome. *Brit. J. Psychiat.* 112:771-778.

95. Clark, D.F. 1970. Behavioral approach to treatment of Gilles de la Tourette's syndrome. *N. Y. St. J. Med.* 70:2205-2210.

96. Claude, H. 1939. Deux etats post-encephalitiques Parkinsonisme, maladie des tics convulsifs avec coprolalie. *Rev. gen. Clin. Ther.* 53:433-434.

97. Clauss, J.L. and Balthasar, K. 1954. Zur kenntnis der generalisierten Tic-Krankheit (Maladie des tics, Gilles de la Tourette'sche Krankheit). *Arch. Psychiat. Nervenkr.* 191:398-418.

98. Colucci, G. 1930. Organic and functional forms of tic. *Rif. Med.* 46:1073-1078.

99. Connell, P.H., Corbett, J.A. and Mathews, A.M. 1967. Drug treatment of adolescent tiqueurs, a double-blind trial of diazepam and haloperidol. *Brit. J. Psychiat.* 113:375-381.

100. Corbett, J.A. 1971. The nature of tics and Gilles de la Tourette's syndrome. *J. psychosom. Res.* 15:403-409.

101. Corbett, J.A., Mathews, A.M., Connell, P.H., and Shapiro, D.A. 1969. Tics and Gilles de la Tourette's syndrome: a follow-up study and critical review. *Brit. J. Psychiat.* 115:1229-1241.

102. Corbett, J.A. 1966. *Paper on childhood tics, delivered to the Child Psychiatry Section of the R.M.P.A.*

103. Corbett, J.A. 1976. In *Gilles de la Tourette's Syndrome.* Ed. F.S. Abuzzahab Sr. and F.O. Anderson. Mason, St. Paul, pp. 3-5; 25-32.

104. Corbett, J.A. 1970. *Tics and the startle response. In press.*

105. Corbin, K.B., Feild, R.J., Goldstein, N.P. and Klass, D.W. 1968. Further observations on Tourette's syndrome. *Aust. Ass. Neurol. Proc.* 5:447-453.

REFERENCES

106. Corbin, K.B. 1970. Common neurophysiologic factors reported in the literature. *N. Y. St. J. Med.* 70:2193-2196.

107. Cornil, L. 1928. Maladie des tics et heredo-syphilis. *Rev. neurol.* 2:17-18.

108. Corning, J.L. 1904-5. Considerations of facial spasm "tic convulsif", mimetic facial spasm. *J. Med. Soc. New Jersey* 1:306-308.

109. Cramer. 1899. Tic convulsivo. *Dtsch. med Wschr.* 25:210.

110. Crane, G.E. 1967. A review of clinical literature on haloperidol. *Int. J. Neuropsychiat.* 3 (suppl#1):110-127.

111. Craven. E.M. 1969. Gilles de la Tourette's syndrome treated with haloperidol. *J. Amer. med. Ass.* 210:134.

112. Creak, M. and Guttman, E. 1935. Chorea, tics and compulsive utterances. *J. ment. Sci.* 81:834-839.

113. Croce, G. 1890. Un caso di tic convulsivo, con ecolalia, coprolalia e melolalia. *Arch. Psichiat.* 11:182-195.

114. Crown, S. 1953. An experimental study into some aspects of the motor behavior and personality of tiqueurs. *J. ment. Sci.* 99:84-91.

115. Cruchet, R. 1906. Sur deux cas de tics convulsifs persistant dans le sommeil. *Rev. neurol.* 14:293-299.

116. Cruchet, R. 1906. Sur un cas de maladie des tics convulsifs. *Arch. gen. Med.* 1:1180-1196.

117. Cruchet, R. 1910. Difficultes du diagnostic entre les crises epileptiques frustes et certains tics convulsifs hysteriques. *Gazz. Hop.* 83:725-730.

118. Cruchet, R. and de Grailly, S. 1923. Tic convulsif hysterique. *Soc. Med. Chir. Bordeaux Bulletins et Memoires,* 484-490.

119. Cukier, M.B. 1949. Kliniczeski syndromy revmaticzeskich porazeni j nerwnoj sistemy. *Zh. Nevropat. Psikhiat.* 18:34-37.

120. Dana, C.L. and Wilkin, W.P. 1886. On convulsive tic with explosive disturbances of speech (so-called Gilles de la Tourette's disease). *J. nerv. ment. Dis.* 11:407-412.

121. Danik, J.J. and Goverdham, M. 1963. Haloperidol in the treatment of 120 psychotic patients. *Amer. J. Psychiat.* 120:389.

REFERENCES

122. Daugela, M.Z. 1961. Psychosomatic tic, a case report with discussion. *Clin. Proc. Child. Hosp. Washington D.C.* 17:235-240.

123. DeGroot, M.H. 1970. A case of Gilles de la Tourette's syndrome occurring in New Zealand. *Aust. N.Z.J. Psychiat.* 4:155-158.

124. Delay, J., Pichot, P., Lemperiere, T. and Elissalde, B. 1960. l'Action du haloperidol dans les psychoses. *Acta. neurol. Belge.* 60:21-38.

125. DeMondragon, C. 1964. Le Traitement des tics par l'haloperidol (R 1625). *Rev. Neuropsychiat. Ouest.* 8:25-31.

126. DeMorsier, G. 1951. Les tics et la maladie des tics convulsifs. *Med. et Hyg.* (Geneve) 9:260:261.

127. Denber, H.C.B., Florio, D., and Rajotte, P. 1962. Third evaluation of haloperidol. *Amer. J. Psychiat.* 119:172-173.

128. DeNigris, G. 1925. Analisi costituzionale e del sistema endocrino-simpatico in un caso de "maladie des tics." *Riv. Sper. Freniat.* 49:309-332.

129. DeRenzi, E. 1892. La malattia del ticchio. *Gazz. Clin.* 3:177-183.

130. D'Errico, A., Sallusto, L. and Tedeschi, G. 1964. Su di un caso di malattia dei tics strattato con talamolisi stereotassica. *Rass. Neuropsichiat.* 18:303-312.

131. Descroizelles. 1890. De quelques cas de tics convulsifs. *Rev. men. Malad. Enfance* 8:337-345.

132. Deshan, P.W. 1961. Gilles de la Tourette's syndrome, report of a case. *J. Oklahoma Med. Ass.* 54:636-638.

133. Desogus, V. 1916. Sulla malattia de Gilles de la Tourette. *Rif. Med.* 32:809-815.

134. Dethlefsen. 1893. Nervesygdomme. *Med. Aarsskr.* 7:68-74.

135. Deutsch, H. 1925. Zur psychogenese eines Ticfalles. *Int. Z. Psychoanal.* 11:325-332.

136. Dewulf, A. and van Bogaert, L. 1940. Etudes anatomo-cliniques de syndromes hypercinetiques complexes. *Mschr. Psychiat. Neurol.* 103:53-61.

137. Deyl, J. 1883. Tic convulsif. *Cas. Lek. ces.* 22:225-243.

138. DiGiacomo, J.N., Fahn, S., Glass, J.B. and Westlake, R.J. 1971. A case with Gilles de la Tourette's syndrome: recurrent refractoriness to haloperidol and unsuccessful treatment with L-dopa. *J. nerv. ment. Dis.* 152:115-117.

139. DiLuzenberger, A. 1897. Tic muscolari semplici, tic emottivi e malattia de Gilles de la Tourette. Naples: *Cav.Dott. vPasquale.*

140. Disertori, B., Granata, M. and Piazza, M. 1967. Contributo ala clinica e terapia della discinesie facciali. *G. Psichiat. Neuropat.* 95:547-564.

141. Divry, P., Bobon, J. and Collard, J. 1960. Rapport sur l'activite neuro-psychopharmacologique du haloperidol (R 1625). *Acta Neurol. Psychiat. Belge.* 60:7-19.

142. Dolmierski, R. and Klossowna, M. 1958. O chorobie Gilles de la Tourette'a. *Neurol. Neurochir. Psychiat. pol.* 8:639-646.

143. Dolmierski, R. and Kloss, M. 1962. De la maladie de Gilles de la Tourette. *Ann. Med.-psychol.* 120:225-232.

144. Domdey, H. 1909. Zur lehre vom Tic general. *Inaug. Diss. Kiel.*

145. Downing, R.W., Comer, N.L. and Ebert, J.N. 1964. Family dynamics in a case of Gilles de la Tourette's syndrome. *J. nerv. ment. Dis.* 138:548-557.

146. Dubois, S. 1901. Traitement des tics convulsifs par la reeducation des centres moteurs. *Bull. gen. Therap.* (Paris) 141:617-627, 142:12-23.

147. Duche, D.J. 1961. Premiers resultats therapeutiques de l'emploi du R 1625 en pedo-psychiatrie. *Rev. neuropsychiat. Hyg. ment. Enf.* 9:288-293.

148. Duffy, R.E. 1950. Tic de Gilles de la Tourette. *Med. Wom. J.* 57:18-21.

149. Dunlap. J.R. 1960. A case of Gilles de la Tourette's disease (maladie des tics): a study of intrafamily dynamics. *J. nerv. ment. Dis.* 130:340-344.

150. Dunlap, J.R. 1945. *Habits: Their Making and Unmaking.* New York: Liveright, p. 195.

151. Eisenberg, L. 1957. Psychiatric implications of brain damage in children. *Psychiat. Quart.* 31:72-92.

152. Eisenberg, L. 1959. Letter in reply to Amer. J. Psychiat. 115:1959, maladie des tics in children. *Amer. J. Psychiat.* 116:178-179.

153. Eisenberg, L., Ascher, E. and Kanner, L. 1959. A clinical study of Gilles de la Tourette's disease (maladie des tics) in children. *Amer. J. Psychiat.* 115:715-723.

154. Ellison, R.M. 1964. Reports of cases, Gilles de la Tourette's syndrome. *Med. J. Aust.* 1:153-155.

155. Emmerich, R. and Loew, O. 1914. Ueber erfolgreiche behandlung des tic convulsif durch chlorkalzium. *Munch. Med. Wschr.* 61:2269-2270.

156. Enoch, D. 1967. *Some uncommon psychiatric syndromes.* Bristol: John Wright & Sons Ltd., pp. 85-97.

157. Erickson, M.H. 1965. Experimental hypnotherapy in Tourette's disease. *Amer. J. clin. Hypnos.* 7:325-331.

158. Eriksson, B. and Persson. T. 1969. Gilles de la Tourette's syndrome, two cases with an organic brain injury. *Brit. J. Psychiat.* 115:351-353.

159. Ey, H. 1948. *Etudes psychiatriques.* Paris.

160. Farber, T. 1885. Uber atypische formen und Kamplikarionen der chorea. *Inaug. Diss.* Berlin.

161. Faux, E.J. 1966. Gilles de la Tourette's syndrome. *Arch. gen. Psychiat.* 14:139-142.

162. Feild, J.R., Corbin, K.B., Goldstein, N.P. and Klass, D.W. 1966. Gilles de la Tourette's syndrome. *Neurology* 16:453-462.

163. Feldman, R.B. and Werry, J.S. 1965. An unsuccessful attempt to treat a tiqueur by massed practice. *Behav. Res. Ther.* 3:111-117.

164. Fenichel, O. 1945. *The psychoanalytic Theory of Neurosis.* New York:Norton.

165. Ferenczi, S. 1926. *Further contributions to the theory and technique of psycho-analysis.* London:Hogarth & The Institute of Psychoanalysis.

166. Ferenczi, S. 1921. Psycho-analytical observations on tic. *Int. J. Psycho-anal.* 2:1-30.

REFERENCES

167. Fernando, S.J.M. 1967. Gilles de la Tourette's syndrome: a report on four cases and a review of published case reports. *Brit. J. Psychiat.* 113:607-617.

168. Fernando, S.J.M. 1968. Gilles de la Tourette's syndrome. *Brit. J. Psychiat.* 114:123-125.

169. Fields, B. 1954. Music as an adjunct in the treatment of brain damaged patients. *Amer. J. Phys. Med.* 33:273-283.

170. Fisarova, M. 1968. Lecba choroby Gilles de la Touretteovy frenolonem. *Bratisl. lek. Listy* 49:670-672.

171. Fisarova, M. 1972. Choroba Gilles de la Touretteova. *Cs. Neurol.* 35:202-208.

172. Fisarova, M. and Kule, J. 1967. Syndrom Gilles de la Tourette. *Cs. Psychiat.* 63:231-235.

173. Fischler. 1905. Ein Fall von generalisierten hysterichen reflextic. *Munch. Med. Wschr.* 52:2540.

174. Flatau, G. 1897. Ueber die Beziehungen zur Tic general und Zwangsvorstellungen. *Zbl. Nervenheilk.* 20:393-395.

175. Ford, C.V. and Gottlieb, F. 1968. A double-blind crossover study of haloperidol in Gilles de la Tourette's syndrome. *Sci. Proc. Amer. Psychiat. Ass.* 124:8-9.

176. Ford, C.V. and Gottlieb, F. 1969. An objective evaluation of haloperidol in Gilles de la Tourette's syndrome. *Dis. nerv. sist.* 30:328-332.

177. Ford, F.R. 1966. *Diseases of nervous system in infancy, childhood and adolescence.* Springfield, Ill.:Thomas.

178. Fourny, L., Segal, J., Combette, H. and Stephanopoli, M.J. 1961. Traitement des accidents aigus de l'alcolisme chronique par le R1625. *Ann Med.-psychol.* 119:991.

179. Fox, W., Gobble, I.F. and Clos, M. 1964. A clinical comparison of trifluperidol, haloperidol and chlorpromazine. *Current Ther. Res.* 6:409-415.

180. Freedman, A.M. and Kaplan, H.I. 1967. Unusual psychiatric disorders, in *Comprehensive Textbooks of Psychiatry.* Baltimore: Williams [c] Wilkins, pp. 1153-1154.

REFERENCES

181. Freud, A. 1946. *The psycho-analytical treatment of children.* New York:International Univ. Press.

182. Friedreich, N. 1881. Ueber coordinierte Erinnerungskrampfe. *Virchows Anat. Psychiol. Med.* 86:430-434.

183. Froste, C.C. 1894. Maladie des tics convulsifs. *Hyg. Med. Farmac. Manadsskrift* 3:201-214.

184. Galvagni, E. 1880. Sugli spasmi ritmici localizzati. *Riv. clin. Bologna* 10:353-359.

185. Gan, A. 1903. Boliezn sudorozhnikh podergivaniy (maladie des tics convulsifs). *Obozr. Psichiat. Nevrol.* 8:38-49.

186. Garry, J.W. and Leonard, T.J. 1962. Haloperidol, a controlled trial in chronic schizophrenia. *J. ment. Sci.* 108:105-107.

187. Geisler, E. 1957. Lokalisierte und generalisierte Tics und ihre Behandlung. *Arch. Kinderheilk.* 155:7-17.

188. Geissman, P., Levy, A. and Israel, L. 1960. Presentation de film, un cas de syndrome Gilles della Tourette. *Ann. Med.-psychol.* 118:578.

189. Gerard, M.W. 1946. The psychogenic tic in ego development. *Psychoanalytical stud. Child* 2:133-162.

190. Gerle, B. 1964. Clinical observations of the side-effects of haloperidol. *Acta paediat. scand.* 40:65-76.

191. Gerle, B., Petersson, B. and Widmark, M. 1961. Kliniska erfarenheler au haldol. *Laekartidnin* 58:1415-1422.

192. Gerstmann, J. and Schilder, P. 1923. Ueber organisch bedingte Tics. *Med. Klin.* 19:896-899.

193. Giberti, F. 1954. Tics multipli e malatti de Gilles de la Tourette, contributi clinic. *Sist. nerv.* 6:136-153.

194. Gilarowski, W.A. 1957. *Psychiatria.* Warszawa:Panstwowy Zaklad Wydawn Lekarskich.

195. Gilbert, M.M. 1969. Haloperidol in severe facial dyskinesia, a case report. *Dis. nerv. Syst.* 30:481-482.

196. Gilles de la Tourette, G. 1881. Les ''sauters'' du Maine (Etats Unis), par G. Beard. *Arch. neurol.* (Paris) 2:146-150.

197. Gilles de la Tourette, G. 1884. Jumping, latah, myriachit. *Arch. neurol.* (Paris) 8:68-84.

198. Gilles de la Tourette, G. 1885. Etude sur une affection nerveuse, caracterisee par de l'incoordination motrice, accompagnee d'echolalie et de coprolalie. *Arch. neurol.* (Paris) 9:19-42, 158-200.

199. Gilles de la Tourette, G. 1899. La maladie des tics convulsifs. *Sem. Med.* (Paris) 19:153-156.

200. Gilles de la Tourette's disease 1958 (note to the editor). *J. Amer. med. Ass.* 151:962-963.

201. Gilmour, A. 1902. Latah among South African natives. *Scot. med. surg. J.* 10:18-20.

202. Grafer, K. 1938. *Zur Frage der maladie des tics.* Dissertation, Munster.

203. Grasset, J. and Rauzier, G. 1890. Lecons sur un cas de maladie des tics et un cas de tremblement singulier de la tete et des membres gauches. *Arch. neurol.* (Paris) 20:27-43, 187-211.

204. Grimaldi, A. 1892. Ipercinesia e psicosi, contributo clinico ala malattia de Gilles de la Tourette o tic convulsivo. *Riv. Psichiat. Neuropat. Med. legale* 1:9-13.

205. Guantieri, G. 1965. l'Ambiente familiare come fattore patogeno: indagine psicosomatica su di un caso gravissimo di malattia dei tics. *Minerva med.* 56:726-729.

206. Guggenheim, P. and Haynal, A. 1964. Uber electroenzephalographische Untersuchungen bei der Maladie Gilles de la Tourette. *Schweiz Arch. Neurol. Neurochir. Pschiat.* 94:265-278.

207. Guinon, G. 1886. Sur la maladie des tics convulsifs. *Rev. Med.* (Paris) 1:50-80.

208. Guinon, G. 1887. Tics convulsifs et hysterie. *Rev. Med.* (Paris) 7:509-519.

209. Gyorgy, L. 1969. Modification of certain central nervous effects of haloperidol during long-term treatment in the mouse and rat. *Psychopharmacologia* (Berl.) 16:223.

210. Habel, A. 1898. Uber Fortbestehen von Tic convulsif bei gleichzeitiger Hemiplegie. *Dtsch. med. Wschr.* 24:189.

211. Hammer, M. 1965. A case of coprolalia in an adolescent boy. *Psychother. Theory Res. Pract.* 2:169-170.

212. Hammond, G.F. 1892. Convulsive tic, its nature and treatment. *Med. Rec.* (N.Y.) 41:236-239.

213. Hammond, W.A. 1884. Myriachit: a newly described disease of the nervous system and its analogues. *Brit. med. J.* 2:758-759.

214. Hassin, G. 1930. Stereotyped acts or attitude tics: a case with a peculiar anomaly of gait. *J. nerv. ment. Dis.* 71:27-32.

215. Healy, C.E. 1970. Gilles de la Tourette's syndrome (maladie des tics), successful treatment with haloperidol. *Amer. J. Dis. Child.* 120:62-63.

216. Healy, N.M. and Fischer, I. 1965. Gilles de la Tourette's syndrome in an autistic child. *J. Irish med. Ass.* 57:93-94.

217. Heigl, F. 1955. Ein Fall von generalisiertem Tic. *Prax. Kinderpsychol.* 4:202-205.

218. Heimlich, E.P. 1965. The specialized use of music as a mode of communication in the treatment of disturbed children. *J. Amer. Acad. Child Psychiat.* 4:86-122.

219. Hengst, E. 1956. Psychotherapeutische Beeinflussung organischer Tic-Erscheinungen. *Psychiat. Neurol. med. Psychol.* (Lpz.) 8:85-87.

220. Heuscher, von J. 1950. Beitrage zur aetiologie der maladie Gilles de la Tourette und zum Regressionsproblem. *Schweiz. Arch. Neurol. Neurochir. Psychiat.* 66:123-158.

221. Heuscher, J.E. 1953. Intermediate states of consciousness in patients with generalized tics. *J. nerv. ment. Dis.* 117:29-38.

222. Heuyer, M., Teysseyre, J., Paupe, M.J. and Martinet, M. 1954. Un cas de tic d'aboiement. *Ann. Med.-psychol.* 112:200-203.

223. Hinsie, L.E. and Campbell, R.J. 1960. *Psychiatric dictionary, 3rd. ed.* New York:Oxford Univ. Press.

224. Hirshfeld, H. 1891. *Uber maladie des tics convulsifs.* Inaugural Dissertation, Berlin.

225. Hoch, P.H. 1945. Neurodynamics of tics. *Nerv. Child* 4:329-334.

226. Hollander, R. 1960. Compulsive cursing, an approach to factors in its genesis, development and pathology. *Psychiat. Quart.* 34:600-622.

227. Holstein, A.P. and Chen, C.H. 1965. Haloperidol, a preliminary clinical study. *Amer. J. Psychiat.* 122:462-463.

228. Hoppe, H.H. 1913. The treatment of tic (myoclonia-paramyoclonia tic, maladie de tic convulsif). *Lancet* 109:649-654.

229. Hunter, W.K. 1898. A case of maladie des tics. *Glasgow med. J.* 1:435-438.

230. Iio, K. and Tange, S. 1963. Tic de Gilles de la Tourette. *Ann. paediat. Jap.* 9:32-36.

231. Infeld, 1898. Verein fur Psychiatrie und Neurologie in Wien. *Wien. klin. Wschr.* 111:17.

232. Itard, J.M.G. 1825. Memoire sur quelques fonctions involontaires des appareils de la locomotion de la prehension et de la voix. *Arch. gen. Med.* 8:385-407.

233. Ivan, L. 1965. A case of Gilles de la Tourette's syndrome, maladie des tics, treated with electroshock therapy. *Int. Cong. Neurol. Proc. Vienna* 8:5-10.

234. Jack, W.R. 1898. Case of maladie des tics. *Glasgow med. J.* 49:266-272.

235. Janssen, P.A.J. 1966. The pharmacological and clinical mode of action of neuroleptic drugs. *Clin. Trials J.* 3:370-379.

236. Johnson, J. 1905. A case of maladie des tic convulsion. *Brit. med. J.* 2:810.

237. Jolly, F. 1892. Ueber die sogenannte Maladie des Tics convulsifs. *Charite-Ann.* 17:740-752.

238. Jones, H.G. 1960. Continuation of Yates' treatment of a tiqueur. In *Behavior Therapy and the Neuroses,* ed. H.J. Eysenck. Oxford: Pergamon.

239. Jouppe, J. 1962. A propos d'un cas de maladie de Gilles de la Tourette. *Ann. Med.-psychol.* 120:147.

240. J. Amer. Med. Ass. 1965. Jumping Frenchmen of Maine. *J. Amer. Med. Ass.* 191:151.

241. Kanner, L. 1957. *Child Psychiatry.* Springfield, Ill. CC. Thomas.

242. Kehrer, F. 1938. Die Verbindung von chorea und ticformigen Hyperkinesien mit Zwangvorstellengen. *Abh. Neurol. Psychiat. Psychol.* 85:7-20.

243. Kelman, D.H. 1965. Gilles de la Tourette's disease in children, a review of the literature. *J. Child psychol.* 6:219-226.

244. Kirillin, A.I. 1899. (Convulsiv tic in a five year old girl.) *Dietskaya Meitsina* 4:411-416. Russian.

245. Klein, M. 1925. Zur Genese des Tics. *Int. Z. Psychoanal.* 11:332.

246. Klemm, R. 1901. *Beitrag zur maladie des tics impulsifs.* Leipzig.

247. Knopp, W. 1967. Tourette's disease. *Int. J. Neuropsychiat.* 105 (suppl#1).

248. Knopp, W. 1970. Man's tripartite brain and psychosomatic medicine. *Psychother. Psychosom.* 18:130-136.

249. Knopp, W. *Psychopathology, anuropathology and electronic pupillography.* To be published.

250. Knopp, W., Strayer, M., Hothem, A. and Furuta, W. 1968. A new approach to an old problem: monitoring the individual response patterns to neuroleptics. *Excerpta med. (Amst.)* Sect. VIII 150:2205-2207.

251. Kodym, O. 1891. Maladie des tics a nektere pribuzne choroby. *Cas. Lek. ces.* 30:163-165.

252. Kolle, K. 1961. *Psychiatrie.* Thieme, Stuttgart.

253. Kopczynski, S. 1900. Przypadek nerwicy ruchowej o charakterze tikow (tics convulsifs) a niezwyklem zaburzeniem mowy. *Gas. Lek. Warszawa* 20:881-885.

254. Koprowska-Milewska, E. 1966. O zespole Gilles de la Tourette's. *Neurol. Neurochir. Psychiat. Pol.* 16:1367-1372.

255. Koster, G. 1899. Ueber die Maladie des Tics impulsifs (mimische Krampfneurose). *Dtsch. Z. Nervenheilk.* 15:147-158.

256. Kovacs, V. 1925. Analyse Eines Falles von tic convulsif. *Int. Z. Psychoanal.* 11:318-325.

REFERENCES

257. Krisch, H. 1930. Zur Theorie der Impuls und Zwangshandlungen. *Z. ges. Neurol. Psychiat.* 130:257-296.

258. Krisch, H. 1930. Die Strukturanalyse der Psychoneurosen (dargestellt an der Hand eines Falles von Tic und generalisiertem Zertrummerungszwang.) *Arch. Psychiat. Nervenkr.* 91:594-95.

259. Kucemilowa, A.P. 1956. Rewmaticzeski j encefalit s hiperkineticzeskim sindromum w detskom wozraste. *Neuropat. Neurochir. Psychiat. Pol.* 56:703-707.

260. Kulovesi, V. 1929. Zur Entstehung des Tics. *Int. Z. Psychoanal.* 15:82-95.

261. Kumento, A. and Koski, M.L. 1967. Syndrome Gilles de la Tourette. *Acta Paediat. scand.* 117(suppl):62-63.

262. Kunkle, E.C. 1965. The "Jumpers" of Maine. *J. Maine med. Ass.* 56:191-193.

263. Kunkle, E.C. 1967. The "Jumpers" of Maine, a reappraisal. *Arch. int. med.* 119:355-358.

264. Kurland, M.L. 1965. Gilles de la Tourette's syndrome: the psychotherapy of two cases. *Comprehens. Psychiat.* 6:298-309.

265. Landis, C., and Hunt, W.A. 1939. *The startle pattern.* New York:Farrar & Rinehart.

266. Langlois, M. and Force, L. 1965. Revision nosologique et clinique de la maladie de Gilles de la Tourette evoquee par l'action de certains neuroleptiques sur son evolution. *Rev. Neurol.* 113:641-645.

267. Latimer, R.H. 1945. The parent-child relationships in children afflicted with tics. *Nerv. Child* 4:353-358.

268. Leclerc, F. and Royer. 1887. Sur un case de spasmes convulsifs et rhythmiques rappelant les cas de pseudo-choree publies sous la rubrique de choree electrique. *Rev. Med.* (Paris) 7:133-136.

269. Legendre, P. 1885. Gilles de la Tourette's syndrome. *St. Louis Courier Med.* 14:275-280.

270. Leger, J.M. and Ranty, Y. 1969. Aspects psychopathologiques de la maladie des tics de Gilles de la Tourette. *Ann. Med.-psychol.* 127:689-695.

REFERENCES

271. Legrain, M. 1889. Deux observations de coprolalie chez les degeneres. *Ann. Med.-psychol.* 2:118-121.

272. Lerch, O. 1901. Convulsive tics. *Amer. med.* 2:694-695.

273. Lewis, A. 1946. Section on psychological medicine. In *Textbook of the Practice of Medicine*, ed. Price. Oxford.

274. Lapolla, A. and Nash, L.R. 1966. A buytrophenone (haloperidol) for the treatment of institutionalized patients. *Int. J. Neuropsychiat.* 2:129.

275. Lett, C.R. 1969. A case of Gilles de la Tourette's disease on active military duty. *Milit. Med.* 134:1445-1446.

276. Levy, B.S. and Ascher, E. 1968. Phenothiazines in the treatment of Gilles de la Tourette's disease. *J. nerv. ment. Dis.* 146:36-40.

277. Levy, D.M. 1944. On the problem of movement restraint. *Amer. J. Orthopsychiat.* 45:644-671.

278. Lewin, K. 1900. Phosphaturie mit Tic convulsif bei einem 3½ jahrigen Kinde. *Arch. Phys-Diat. Ther.* 2:281-2.

279. Lindner, H. 1967. Hypnotherapy and psychodynamics in the syndrome of Gilles de la Tourette. *Int. J. clin. exp. Hypnos.* 15:151-155.

280. Lorand, B. 1949. Les tics nerveux des enfants. *Paed. Denubiana-* 6:203-230.

281. Lorenzetti, E. 1903. A proposito di alcuni casi di tic convulsivo. *Gazz. Osp. Clin.* 140:1478-1481.

282. Lucas, A.R. 1964. Gilles de la Tourette's disease in children: treatment with phenothiazine drugs. *Amer. J. Psychiat.* 121:606-608.

283. Lucas, A.R. 1966. Psychopharmacological treatment. In *The Psychiatric Disorders of Childhood*, ed. C.R. Shaw, New York:Appleton-Century-Crofts, Ch. 19.

284. Lucas, A.R. 1967. Gilles de la Tourette's disease in children: treatment with haloperidol. *Amer. J. Psychiat.* 124:146-49.

285. Lucas, A.R., Kaufmann, P.E., and Morris, E.M. 1967. Gilles de la Tourette's disease: a clinical study of 15 cases. *J. Amer. Acad. Child Psychiat.* 6:700-722.

REFERENCES

286. Lucas, A.R. 1970. Gilles de la Tourette's disease: an overview. *N.Y. St. J. Med.*70:2197-2200.

287. Lucas, A.R. and Rodin, E.A. 1973. The EEG in Gilles de la Tourette's disease. *Dis. nerv. Syst.* 34:85-89.

288. Lyon, E. 1923. Die psychopathische Grundlage zum tic bie Kindern.*Z. Kinderforsch.* 28:64-70.

289. MacDonald, I.J. 1963. A case of Gilles de la Tourette's syndrome, with some aetiological observations. *Brit. J. Psychiat.* 109:206-210.

290. MacFarlane, J.W. 1954. In *Behaviour problems of normal children.* California: University of California Publications in Child Development.

291. Mack, E.G. 1921. Notes on a case of multiple tics. *J. Ceylon Br. Brit. med. Ass.* 18:23.

292. Maffei, G., Pogglali, B., Pescetto, G. 1965. Tics e depersonalizzazione. *Riv. Neurobiol.* 9:190-196.

293. Magowska, I. and Szafranek, J. 1965. Przypadek choroby Gilles de la Tourette. *Neurol. Neurochir. Psychiat. pol.* 15:937-939.

294. Mahler, M.S. 1944. Tics and impulsions in children: a study of motility. *Psychoanal. Quart.* 13:430-455.

295. Mahler, M.S. 1945. Introductory remarks. *Nerv. Child* 4:307.

296. Mahler, M.S. 1949. Psychoanalytic evaluation of tic in psychopathology of children, in the *Psychoanalytic Study of the Child.* New York:International Univ. Press, pp. 279-307.

297. Mahler, M.S. and Rangell, L. 1943. A psychosomatic study of maladie des tics (Gilles de la Tourette's disease). *Psychiat. Quart.* 17:579-603.

298. Mahler, M.S. and Gross, I.H. 1945. Psychotherapeutic study of a typical case with tic syndrome. *Nerv. Child* 4:359-373.

299. Mahler, M.S., Luke, J.A. and Daltroff, W. 1945. Clinical and follow-up study of the tic syndrome in children. *Amer. J. Orthopsychiat.* 15:631-647.

300. Mahler, M.S. and Luke, J.A. 1946. Outcome of the tic syndrome. *J. nerv. ment. Dis.* 103:433-445.

REFERENCES

301. Malattia dei tics e corea di Sydenham, 1899. *Gazz. Osp. Milan* 30:1321-1323.

302. Mannini, C. 1902. Coree, policloni, tic e malattia dei tic. *Rif. Med.* 3:137-139.

303. Marchand, L. 1909. Maladie de Gilles de la Tourette et paralysie general. *Rev. neurol.* 17:659-662.

304. Mari, A. 1929. Tic postencefalitico insolito. *Riv. Pat. nerv. ment.* 34:282-287.

305. Martin, J.P. and Hurwitz, L.J. 1962. Locomotion and the basal ganglia. *Brain* 85:261-277.

306. Matheson, A.R. 1898. A case of Gilles de la Tourette's disease. *Methodist Episcopal Hospital Report* 1:381-383.

307. Mathews, A.M., Corbett, J.A. and Connell, P.M. *Treatment of tics and Gilles de la Tourette's syndrome with haloperidol.* In preparation.

308. Mattson, R.H. and Calverly, J.R. 1968. Dextroamphetamine sulfate-induced dyskinesias. *J. Amer. med. Ass.* 204:400-402.

309. Maugeri, F.T. 1911. Malattia di Gilles de la Tourette. *Policlinico, Sez. Med.* 18:1040-1041.

310. Mazur. W.P. 1953. Gilles de la Tourette's syndrome. *Edinb. med. J.* 60:427-433.

311. Mazur, W.P. Gilles de la Tourette's syndrome. *Canadian med. Ass. J.* 69:520-522.

312. McKinnon, R.C. 1967. Gilles de la Tourette's syndrome: a case showing electroencephalographic changes and response to haloperidol. *Med. J. Aust.* 54:21-22.

313. Medical World News: Taming a tic with tranquilizer. *Med. Wld. News*, February 25, 1972, p. 29.

314. Meige, H. and Feindel, E. 1901. Sur la curabilite des tics. *Gazz. Hop.* 74:673-677.

315. Meige, H. and Feindel, E. 1901. l'Etat mental des tiqueurs. *Rev. Neurol.* 9:785-786.

REFERENCES

316. Meige, H. and Feindel, E. 1907. *Tics and their treatment.* Tr. and ed. S.A.K. Wilson. New York: William Wood & Co.

317. Menaker, E. 1945. Hypermotility and transitory tic in a child of seven. *Nerv. Child.* 4:335-341.

318. Mesnikoff, A.M. 1959. Three cases of Gilles de la Tourette's syndrome treated with psychotherapy and chlorpromazine. *Arch. Neurol. Psychiat.* (Chic.) 81:710.

319. Messiha, F.S., Knopp, W., Vanecko, S., O'Brien, V. and Corson, S.A. 1971. Haloperidol therapy in Tourette's syndrome: neurophysiological, biochemical and behavioral correlates. *Life Sci.* 10:449-457.

320. Meurice, E. 1960. Etude electroencephalographique du R.-1625. *Acta neurol. belg.* 60:91-95.

321. Meyer. 1914. Psychogen bedingte an Maladie des Tics erinnernde Zuckungen. *Dtsch. med. Wschr.* 40:467.

322. Michael, R.P. 1957. Treatment of a case of compulsive swearing. *Brit. med. J.* 1:1506-1508.

323. Mignard. 1909. Apparition de tics et de phenomenes convulsifs lies a un delire melancholique chez une degeneree hereditaire. *Rev. Psychiat.* 13:97-102.

324. Milman, D.H. 1960. Multiple tics. *Amer. J. Psychiat.* 116:935-936.

325. Mirto, G. 1890. La malattia dei tic convulsivi. *G. Neuropat.* 7:248-264.

326. Mitchell, S.D. and Zanker, A. 1948. Use of music in group therapy. *J. ment. Sci.* 94:737-748.

327. Mittelman, B. 1958. Psychodynamics of motility. *Int. J. Psycho-anal.* 39:196-199.

328. Moldofsky, H. 1971. A psychophysiological study of multiple tics. *Arch. gen. Psychiat.* 25:79-87.

329. Monnerot, E., Chancel, M. and Danjard, J. 1961. Notes therapeutiques sur l'association d'entree et constante d'un neuroleptique majeur le R-1625 avec un anti-parkinsonien le 2987 RP. *Ann. Med.-psychol.* 119:669-704.

330. Monnier, M., Sauer, R. and Hait, A.M. 1970. The activating effect of histamine on the central nervous system. *Int. Rev. Neurobiol.* 12:265-305.

331. Morell, H. 1903. General convulsive tic with coprolalia. *Med. News* (N.Y.) 83:1082-1083.

332. Morphew, J.A. and Sim, M. 1969. Gilles de la Tourette's syndrome: a clinical and psychopathological study. *Brit. J. med. Psychol.* 4:293-301.

333. Mouren, P., Berthon, M., Pache, R. and Alliez, J. 1964. Maladie des tics associee a un nervose obsessionnelle severe. *Ann. Med.-psychol.* 122:821.

334. Moyer, H.N. 1897. A case of tic convulsif. *Chicago med. Recorder* 8:27-28.

335. Muller, O. 1889. *Uber die als maladie des tics beschriebene Krankheit.* Inaugural Dissertation, Berlin.

336. Nada Raja, R. 1970. Letter to the editor. *Brit. J. Psychiat.* 117:476.

337. Naumburg, M. 1945. The psychodynamics of the art expression of a boy patient with tic syndrome. *Nerv. Child* 4:374-409.

338. Negro, D.C. 1909. Un caso di malattia de Gilles de la Tourette. *Riv. Neuropat.* 3:346-352.

339. Newmark, L. 1894. Ein fall von Maladie des tics convulsifs. *Festschrift zum 25th Jubilaeum des Vereins Deutscher Aerzte,* San Francisco, Cal. pp. 29-32.

340. Nogues, M.E. 1902. Des tics en general. *Rev. Neurol.* 10:766-798.

341. Noir, J. 1893. *Etude sur les tics.* Paris:Bureaux du Progres Medical.

342. Noiszewski, K. 1904. Przyczynek do powstawania i leczenia tic convulsif. *Now. Lek.* 16:493-494.

343. Nordoff, P. and Robbins, C. 1965. *Music Therapy for Handicapped Children.* Blauvelt, N.Y.:Rudolph Steiner Pbns.

344. North, R.R. 1971. Drug induced movement disorders. *Postgrad. Med.* 50:180-185.

345. Nylander, I. 1951. Application of protracted sleep in treatment of difficult tics. *Acta paedopsychiat.* 18:167-173.

346. O'Brien, J.A. 1884. Jumping, latah, myriachit. *Arch. neurol.* (Chic.) 8:68.

347. O'Brien, M.A. 1883. Latah. *J. Brit. Asiat. Soc.* 1:381.

348. Oddo, C. 1899. Le diagnostic differentiel de la maladie des tics et de la choree de Sydenham. *Presse med.* 7:189-191.

349. Oettinger, B. 1899. The disease of convulsive tic (Gilles de la Tourette's disease). *Amer. J. med. Sci.* 118:303-312.

350. Olivennes, M. 1970. Maladie des tics. *Ann. Pediat.* 17:911-914.

351. Oppenheim, H. 1887. Eine seltene Motilitatsneurose. *Berl. klin. Wschr.* 24:309.

352. Oppenheim, H. 1902. Bemerkungen zur Lehre vom Tic. *J. Psychol. Neurol.* (Lpz.) 1:139-146.

353. Oppolzer. 1861. Krampf des Gesichtsnerven, tic convulsif. *Allg. Wien. med. Z.* 10:73.

354. Osetowska, E. 1966. Quatre cas d'encephalite dite rhumatismale. *Neuropath. pol.* 4(suppl):751-758.

355. Osler, W. 1891. *On chorea and choreiform affections.* London:H.K. Lewis.

356. Osler, W. 1890. On the form of convulsive tic associated with coprolalia. *Med. News* (N.Y.) 27:645-647.

357. Pacella, B.L. 1945. Physiologic and differential diagnostic considerations of tic manifestations in children. *Nerv. Child* 4:313-317.

358. Paley, H.M., Harkoff, L.D., Kawi, A.A. and Mendelsohn, F.S. 1962. A preliminary study of a butyrophenone derivative in inpatients and outpatients. *J. Neuropsychiat.* 4:39-42.

359. Pasamanick, B., and Kawi, A. 1956. A study of the association of prenatal and paranatal factors with the development of tics in children. *J. Paediat.* 48:596-601.

360. Pastena, A. 1901. Contributo clinico alla malattia Gilles de la Tourette. *Incurabili* 16:15-44.

361. Paterson, M.T. 1945. Spasmodic torticollis, results of psychotherapy in 21 cases. *Lancet* 2:556-559.

362. Patrick, H.T. 1905. Convulsive tic. *J. Amer. med. Ass.* 44:437-442.

363. Patrick, H.T. 1909. Remarks on tic and chorea. *J. Amer. med. Assoc.* 52:1373-1375.

364. Paul, R. and Staudt, V.M. 1953. Music therapy for the mentally ill, a historical sketch. *J. gen. Psychol.* 59:167-178.

365. Paulian, D. and Bistriceano, I. 1923. Tics multiples d'origine professionelle. *Encephale* 18:660.

366. Pautyrikhoff, J.I. 1886. (A case of imitative disease.) *Russ. Med.* 2:193. Russian.

367. Peck, M.W. 1923. Two cases of major tic. *J. nerv. ment. Dis.* 58:297-308.

368. Perini, U. and Lampo, B. 1964. l'Haloperidol nella terapia delle sindromi ticcose. *Minerva med.* 55:3387-3390.

369. Piotrowski, Z.A. 1945. Rorschach records of children with tic syndrome. *Nerv. Child* 4:342-352.

370. Pitres, A. 1901. Tics convulsifs generalises traites et gueris par la gymnastique respiratoire. *J. Med. Bordeaux* 31:106-108.

371. Plavec, V. 1904. Tic convulsif. *Wien. med. Presse* 45:1621, 1667, 1706, 1754.

372. Polites, D.J., Kruger, D. and Stevenson, I. 1965. Sequential treatments in a case of Gilles de la Tourette's syndrome. *Brit. J. med. Psychiat.* 38:43-52.

373. Pope, C. 1928. Motor tics. *Med. J. Rec.* 127:436-439.

374. Prabhakaran, N. 1970. A case of Gilles de la Tourette's syndrome with some observations on etiology and treatment. *Brit. J. Psychiat.* 116:539-541.

375. Pratt, J.P., Bishop, M.P. and Gallant, D.M. 1964. Comparison of haloperidol, trifluperidol and chlorpromazine in acute schizophrenic patients. *Current ther. Res.* 6:562-571.

REFERENCES

376. Prince, M. 1906. Case of multiform tic including automatic speech and purposive movements. *J. nerv. ment. Dis.* 33:29-34.

377. Pringle, M.L., Bulter, N.R. and Davie, R. 1967. *11,000 Seven Year Olds.* London: National Bureau for Cooperation in Child Care, p. 185.

378. Prot, J. 1959. Przypadek zespolu Gilles de la Tourette'a. *Neurol. Neurochir. Psychiat.* pol. 9:639-644.

379. Rafi, A.A. 1962. Learning theory and the treatment of tics. *J. Psychosom. Res.* 6:71-76.

380. Railton, T.C. 1886. Notes of a case of involuntary muscular movements accompanied by coprolalia. *Med. Chron.* 4:24-29.

381. Randrup, A. and Munkvad, I.D. 1969. Pharmacological studies on the brain mechanisms underlying two forms of behavioral excitation: stereotyped hyperactivity and "rage". *Ann. N.Y. Acad. Sci.* 159:928-938.

382. Ranty, Y. 1970. *l'Aspect phychiatrique de la maladie des tics de Gilles de la Tourette.* Dissertation, Bordeaux.

383. Rapoport, J. 1959. Maladie des tics in children. *Amer. J. Psychiat.* 116:177-178.

384. Raymond. 1901. Maladie des tics avec coprolalie. *Rev. Hypn. Psychol. Physiol.* 16:126.

385. Raymond. 1910. Maladie des tics. *Med. Mod.* 21:393.

386. Reich, W. 1924-5. Der psychogene tic als Onanie-equivalent. *Z. Sexualwissenschaft* 11:302-313.

387. Remouchamps, E. 1895. Sur les troubles mentaux dans la maladie des tics convulsifs. *Bull. Soc. Med. ment. belg.* pp. 24-32.

388. Remouchamps, E. 1895. Bijdrage tot de kennis der neurose, bekend onder den naam van "maladie des tics convulsifs." *Nederl. T. Geneesk* part 1 31:539-543.

389. Ritvo, S. 1944-5. Survey of the recent literature on tics in children. *Nerv. Child* 4:308-312.

390. Robinson, R.J. 1966. Gilles de la Tourette's disease. *Develop. Med. Child Neurol.* 8:599-612.

REFERENCES

391. Rodenberg, L. 1962. Psychische Faktoren bei einegen motorische Storungen. *Z. psychosom. Med. psychoanal.* 8:77-94.

392. Rosenheim, F. 1948. Animal identifications in a tiqueur. *Amer. J. Orthopsychiat.* 18:529-535.

393. Ross, T.W.E. 1909. A case of convulsive tic. *Brit. med. J.* 2:135-316.

394. Roubinovitch, J. 1892. Sur un cas de maladie des tics convulsifs avec mouvement par obsession. *Ann. Med.-psychol.* 16:467-477.

395. Roubinovitch, J. 1906. Iconographie de l'evolution d'un cas de maladie des tics. *Nuovo Iconogr. Salpetriere* 19:289-292.

396. Roumojan, U. 1957. Un cas de psychotherapie psychoanalytique instituee pour des tics. *Rev. franc. Psychoanal.* 21:707-713.

397. Runge, W. 1932. Beitrag zum Ticproblem. *Dtsch. Z. Nervenheilk.* 127:96-115.

398. Rutter, M., Lebovici, S., Eisenberg, L., Sneznevskij, A.V., Saudoun, R., Brooke, E. and Yi Lin, T. 1969. A tri-axial classification of mental disorders in childhood. *Child. Psychol. Psychiat.* 10:41-61.

399. Rutter, M., Tizard, J. and Whitmore, K. 1970. In *Health, Education and Behavior.* London:Longmans.

400. Sala, E. 1956. La malattia di Gilles de la Tourette. *Ann. Neuropsichiat. Psicoanal.* 3:559-588.

401. Salmi, K. 1961. Gilles de la Tourette's disease, the report of a case and its treatment. *Acta Psychiat. scand.* 36:157-162.

402. von Sarbo, A. 1901. Maladie des tics und die damit in Verbindung stehenden Sprachstoerungen. *Med. Paed. Mschr. ges. Spracheilk* 19:205-210.

403. Soroja Bai, B.K. 1966. An interesting case report on Gilles de la Tourette's disease. *Indian J. Psychiat.* 8:228-232.

404. Sarteschi, P. 1956. Sulla delimitazione de la malattia de Gilles de la Tourette. *Rass. Studi. Psychiat.* 45:960-970.

405. Savill, T.D. 1907. Two cases of convulsive tic affecting the respiratory muscles and the upper extremities, in both of which the condition had existed more or less for ten years. *Proc. neurol. Soc. London* 30:150-151.

REFERENCES

406. Savill, T.D. 1909-10. Three cases of spasmodic tic. *Trans. med. Soc. London* 33:331-334.

407. Savin, L.H. 1962. Remarks on spasms and tics in ophthalmic practice with notes of four cases of the syndrome of Gilles de la Tourette. *Trans. ophthal. Soc. U.K.* 81:39-52.

408. Schilder, P. 1940. The structure of obsessions and compulsions. *Psychiatry* 3:549-560.

409. Schlesinger. 1892. Wiener medizinischer Club presentation. *Neurol. Cbl.* 11:761.

410. Schneck, J.M. 1960. Gilles de la Tourette's disease. *Amer. J. Psychiat.* 117:78.

411. Schneider, D.E. 1938. The clinical syndromes of echolalia, echopraxia, grasping and sucking. *J. nerv. ment. Dis.* 88:18-35, 88:200-216.

412. Sciamanna, E. 1897. Sulla malattia dei tic. *Riv. Quindicinal Psicol. Psichiat. Neuropath.* 1:243-248, 257-264.

413. Seglas, J. 1888. Quelques considerations sur l'etat mental dans les chorees. *Soc. Med. ment. Belg.* 51:342-354.

414. Seglas, J. 1888. Quelques considerations sur l'etat mental dans les chorees. *Soc. Med. ment. belg.* 51:342-354.

415. Seignot, J.N. 1961. Un cas de maladie des tics de Gilles de la Tourette gueri par le R-1625. *Ann. Med.-psychol.* 119:578-579.

416. Selling, L. 1929. Infection in the etiology of tics. *Arch. Neurol. Psychiat.* 22:1163.

417. Shapiro, A.K. 1970. Dangers of premature psychologic diagnosis. *N.Y. St. J. Med.* 70:2210-2214.

418. Shapiro, A.K. 1970. Gilles de la Tourette's syndrome. *N.Y. St. J. Med.* 70:2193.

419. Shapiro, A.K. and Shapiro, E. 1968. Treatment of Gilles de la Tourette's syndrome with haloperidol. *Brit. J. Psychiat.* 114:345-350.

420. Shapiro, A.K. and Shapiro, E. 1971. Clinical dangers of psychological theorizing, Gilles de la Tourette's syndrome. *Psychiat. Quart.* 45:159-171.

421. Shirakawa, T., Inoue, K. and Inenaga, K. 1969. (A diagnostically difficult case manifesting facial tic and mutism.) *Clin. Neurol.* 9:156. Japanese.

422. Shkarin, A.N. 1903. K Kazuistiki tic convulsif v dietskom vozrastie. *Sovetsk Vrach. Gaz.* 10:535.

423. Siebert, C. 1896. Ein Fall von Maladie des tics convulsifs mit Athetosebewegungen. *Dtsch. med. Wschr.* 22:808-809.

424. Sievert, C. 1913. *Casuistischer Beitrag zur Lehre von der maladie des tics convulsifs.* Inaugural Dissertation, Dulmen.

425. Silbiger, B. 1928. Zur Frage der Mitbewegungen und Tics. *Med. Klin.* 1:654.

426. Singer, K. 1963. Gilles de la Tourette's disease. *Amer. J. Psychiat.* 120:80-81.

427. Singer, K. 1970. Gilles de la Tourette's syndrome. *Brit. J. Psychiat.* 117:476-477.

428. Slap, J.W. 1957. Psychotherapy with a case of maladie des tics. *N.Y. Hillside Hosp. J.* 6:43-54.

429. Smith, C.G. 1969. Gilles de la Tourette syndrome treated with LSD. *Irish J. med Sci.* 2:269-271.

430. Snyder, S.H., Taylor, K.M., Coyle, J.T. and Meyerhoff, J.L. 1970. The role of brain dopamine in behavioral regulation and the actions of psychotropic drugs. *Amer. J. Psychiat.* 127:199-207.

431. Sobieski, T. 1964. A propos de la maladie de Gilles de la Tourette. *Sem. ther.* 40:129.

432. Spehl, E. 1899. A propos du traitement de la maladie des tics. *J. belge Neurol. Psychiat.* 4:289-291.

433. Stanciu, E., Csiky, K. and Csiky, C.S. 1972. Observatii asupra unui cas de boala ticurilor (Sindromul Gilles de la Tourette) tratat cu haloperidol. *Neurol. Psihiat. Neurochir.* 17:43-48.

434. Steenfeldt-Foss, O.W. 1963. Kliniske Erfaringer med Haloperidol Behandlung av Langtidspasienter. *Tidskr. norske Laegeforen.* 83:1038-1041.

435. Stembo, L. 1891. Ein Fall von Gilles de la Tourette'scher Krankheit. *Berl. klin. Wschr.* 28:697-699.

436. Stengel, E. 1945. Study on some clinical aspects of relationship between obsessional neurosis and psychotic reaction types. *J. ment. Sci.* 91:166-187.

437. Stengel, E. 1947. A clinical and psychological study of echo-reactions. *J. ment. Sci.* 93:598-612.

438. Stevens, H. 1965. Jumping Frenchmen of Maine (myriachit). *Arch. Neurol.* (Chic.) 12:311-314. (Trans. *Amer. Neurol. Ass.* 89:65-67, 1964).

439. Stevens, H. 1971. Gilles de la Tourette and his syndrome by serendipity. *Amer. J. Psychiat.* 128:489-492.

440. Stevens, H. 1964. The syndrome of Gilles de la Tourette and its treatment. *Med. Ann. D.C.* 33:277-279.

441. Stevens, J.R. and Blachly, P.H. 1966. Successful treatment of the maladie des tics. *Amer. J. dis. Child.* 112:541-545.

442. Stiefler, G. 1935. Uber die tics. *Wien. klin. Wschr.* 48:1439-1443.

443. Stiefler, G. 1936. Tics. In *Handbuch der Neurologie,* ed Bumke and Foerster, Berlin:Springer, p. 1046.

444. Straus, E. 1927. Uber die organische Natur der Tics und der Koprolalie. *Zbl. ges. Neurol.* 47:698-699.

445. Straus, E. 1927. Untersuchungen uber die postchoreatischen Motilitatsstorungen, insbesondere die Beziehungen der Chorea minor zum Tic. *Mschr. J. Psychiat. Neurol.* 66:261, 294-299.

446. Subramaniam, M. 1966. The Gilles de la Tourette syndrome. *Med. J. Malaya* 21:95-96.

447. Sulestrowska, H. 1967. Tiki Tourette'a z zespolem anankastycznym i charakteropatia u dziecka. *Psychiat. pol.* 1:375-379.

448. Sulestrowski, W. and Wdowiak, L. 1957. O uwarunkowanych organicznie zespolach nerwicowych. *Pol. Tyg. Lek.* 4:1524-1528.

449. Takehashi, G. 1901. (Maladie des tics convulsifs.) *Chiugai Iji Shinpo* 22:365-368. Japanese.

450. Tapia, F. 1969. Haldol in the treatment of children with tics and stutterers, and an incidental finding. *Psychiat. Quart.* 43:647-649.

451. Thomas. 1901. Contribution a l'etude de la maladie des tics chez l'infant. *Gazz. Malad. Infant* 3:337.

452. Tobin, W.G. and Reinhart, J.B. 1961. Tics de Gilles de la Tourette. *Amer. J. Dis. Childr.* 101:778-783.

453. Tokarsky, A.A. 1890. Meriatschenje und Maladie des Tics convulsifs. *Neurol. Cbl.* 9:663.

454. Tokarsky, A.A. 1893. Meryacheniye i boliezn sudorozhnikh podergivaniy. Moscow:Richter.

455. Tokarksy, A.A. 1893. Uber die Maladie des tics convulsifs. *Neurol. Cbl.* 12:565.

456. Toporkov. N. and Zykova, L.Y. 1933. (Relation of congenital syphilis to convulsive tic.) *Sovetsk. klin.* 19:356. (Russian).

457. Torup, E. 1962. A follow-up study of children with tics. *Acta Paediat.* 51:261-268.

458. Trousseau. 1873. *Clinique medical de l'hotel Dieu de Paris.* 2:267.

459. Ungher, J., Ciurea, E. and Volanschi, D. 1962. Electroencephalographic analysis of motor neurosis in children (infantile tics). *Electroenceph. Clin. Neurophysiol.* 14:147.

460. Van Bogaert, L. 1947. La methode histologique et les problemes de maladie de la substance blanche. *J. belge. Neurol. Psychiat.* 47:82-110.

461. Van Bogaert, L., Radermacker, J. and Titeca, J. 1950. Les syndromes myocloniques. *Neurol. psych.* 953:650-690.

462. Van Brero, P.C.Z. 1895. Ueber das sogenannte Latah ein in Niederlandisch-Ostindien verkommende Neurose. *Allg. Z. Psychiat. Psychisch-Gericht. Med.* 51:939-948.

463. Von Dishoek, H.A.E. and Stekel, W. 1922. Die psychisch Behandlung des Tic. *Ther. d. Genenw.* 63:296-308.

464. Van Gehuchten. 1899. Un curieux cas de tic. *J. belge Neurol.* 4:48-51.

REFERENCES

465. Vencovsky, E. and Fisarova, M. 1969. Die Anwedung von Frenolon bei der Behandlung des Tics. *Arzneimittal-Forsch.* 19:518.

466. Vizioli, R. 1893. Un caso di tic convulsivo con ecolalia e coprolalia. *Lavori Cong. Med. Intern.* 5:479, 482.

467. Vizioli, R. 1897. Un caso di tic convulsivo. *Boll. clin.* 14:193-197.

468. Von Gorlitzer von Mundy. 1947. Uber tic convulsive und sein Behandlung. *Klin. Med. (Wien.)* 20:984-988.

469. Waelkens, J. 1960. Etude clinique du R-1625 (Haloperidol). *Acta neurol. belg.* 60:128-134.

470. Wagner, E.E. 1970. Results of psychological testing on a child with Gilles de la Tourette's disease. *J. clin. Psychol.* 26:52-57.

471. Wall Street Journal. 1972. Rare illness reduces victims to shouts, grunts — and swearing, reported by Barry Kramer. *Wall Street J.* June 20, 1972, p. 1.

472. Wallin, C.C. 1904. General tic, with report of a case. *J. Mich. med. Soc.* 3:479-486.

473. Walsh, PJ.F. 1962. Compulsive shouting and Gilles de la Tourette's disease. *Brit. J. clin. Pract.* 16:651-655.

474. Walther, K. 1950. Falle von Tic general. *Zbl. ges. Neurol.* 3:286.

475. Walton, D. 1961. Experimental psychology and the treatment of a tiqueur. *J. Child Psychol.* 2:148-155.

476. Wanke, R. 1947. Zur Behandlung des mimischen Gesichtskrampfes. *Chirurg.* 17-18:640-648.

477. Weingarten, K. 1968. Einige Bemarkungen zum Ticproblem. *Wien. klin. Wschr.* 80:83-87.

478. Weisman, A.D. 1952. Nature and treatment of tics in adults. *Arch. Neurol. Psychiat* (Chic.) 68:444.

479. Wesolowski, L. 1968. *Psychiat. pol.* 5:597-598.

480. Whatmore, G.B. 1962. A neurophysiologic view of functional disorders. *Psychosomatics* 3:371-378.

REFERENCES

481. Wilder, J. 1928. Neure Erkenntnisse zur Pathogenese und Therapie des Tic convulsif. *Wien. med. Wschr.* 78:949-951.

482. Wilder, J. 1930. Der tic convulsif. *Jbr. arztl. Fortbild.* 21:13-27.

483. Wilder, J. 1946. Tic convulsif as a psychosomatic problem. *Nerv. Child.* 5:265-371.

484. Wilder, J. and Silbermann, I. 1927. Ein Fall von Maladie des tics. *Neurol. Psychiat.* 43:1.

485. Wilder, J. and Silbermann, I. 1927. *Beitrage zum ticproblem.* Berlin: Karger.

486. Wille, H. 1898. Ueber einen Fall von Maladie des tics impulsifs (Gilles de la Tourette'sche Krankheit). *Mschr. Psychiat. Neurol.* 4:210-226.

487. Wilson, J.C. 1897. A case of tic convulsif (maladie des tics). *Arch. Pediat.* 14:881-887.

488. Wilson, S.A.K. 1927. The tics and allied conditions. *J. Neurol. Psychopath.* 8:93-109.

489. Wilson, S.A.K. 1955. Motor neuroses. In *Neurology*, 2nd ed., ed. A.N. Bruce, Baltimore:Williams & Wilkins, vol. 3, pp. 1921-1927.

490. Wohlfahrt, G., Ingvar, D.H. and Hellberg, A.M. 1961. Compulsive shouting (Benedek's "klazomania") associated with oculogyric spasms in chronic epidemic encephalitis. *Acta psychiat. scand.* 36:369-377.

491. Wolffenbuttel, E. 1963. (Neurotic defensive syndromes.) *Rev. bras. Med.* 20:363-364. Portuguese.

492. Yap, P.M. 1952. The latah reaction, its pathodynamics and nosological position. *J. ment. Sci.* 98:516-564.

493. Yates, A.J. 1958. The application of learning theory to the treatment of tics. *J. Abnorm. soc. Psychol.* 56:175-182.

494. Yvonneau, M. and Beard, P. 1970. Sur un cas de maladie des tics bloquee par le sulpiride. *Encephale* 59:439-459.

495. Zausmer, D.M. 1954. Treatment of tics in childhood. *Arch. Dis. Childr.* 29:537-542.

496. Zgirski, L. 1968. Przypadek ptyzeomanii w zespole Gilles de la Tourette'a. *Psychiat. pol.* 2:95-98.

497. Zimmerman, E.K.W. 1958. Intrakutane Behandlung eines Falles von Tic convulsif. *Hippokrates* (Stuttg.) 29:600.

498. Znamierowska-Kozik, M. and Gasiorowska, B. 1966. Obraz elektroencefalograficzny w przypadkach tikow u dzieci. *Neurol. Neurochir. Psychiat. pol.* 16:583-588.

Addendum to Gilles de la Tourette's Bibliography:

499. Meyerhoff, J.L. and Snyder, S.H. 1973. Gilles de la Tourette's disease and minimal brain dysfunction: Amphetamine isomers reveal catecholamine correlates in an affected patient. *Psychopharmacologia,* 29:211-220.

500. Shapiro, A.K., Shapiro, E. and Wayne, H. 1972. Birth, developmental and family histories, and demographic information in Tourette's syndrome. *J. Nerv. ment. Dis.* 155:335-344.

501. Shapiro, A.K., Shapiro, E. and Wayne, H. 1973. The symptomatology and diagnosis of Gilles de la Tourette's Syndrome. *J. am. Acad. child Psychiat.* 12:702-723.

502. Shapiro, A.K., Shapiro, E. and Wayne, H. 1973. The treatment of Gilles de la Tourette's syndrome with haloperidol: Review of 34 cases. *Arch. gen. Psychiat.* 28:92-97.

503. Shapiro, A.K., Shapiro, E., Wayne, H. and Clarkin, J. 1972. The psychopathology of Gilles de la Tourette's syndrome. *Am. J. Psychiat.* 129:427-34.

504. Shapiro, A.K., Shapiro, E., Wayne, H. and Clarkin, J. *Organic factors in Gilles de la Tourette's syndrome.* In press.

505. Shapiro, A.K., Shapiro, E., Wayne, H., Clarkin, J. and Bruun, R.D. 1973. Tourette's syndrome: Summary of data on 34 patients. *Psych. som. Med.* 35:419-434.

506. Shapiro, E., Shapiro, A.K. and Clarkin, J. *Clinical psychological testing in Tourette's syndrome.* In press.

507. Sweet, R.D., Solomon, G.E., Wayne, H., Shapiro, E., Shapiro, A.K. *Neurologic features of Gilles de la Tourette's syndrome.* In press.

508. Wayne, H., Shapiro, A.K. and Shapiro, E. 1972. Gilles de la Tourette's syndrome: Electroencephalographic investigation and clinical correlation. *J. clin. Electroencephalogr.* 3:160-168.

INDEX

INDEX